Superhero Moms, Warrior Kids

Stories of Love, Strength, and Triumph Raising Type 1 Kids

Erin Hayden

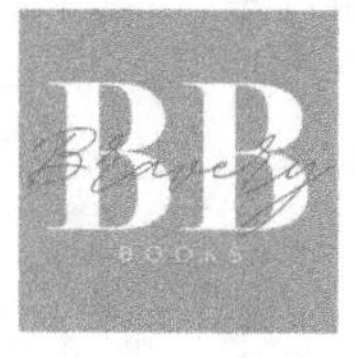

Bravery Books

Dedication

Dedication

This book is dedicated in loving memory of James Hayden, a beloved father and grandfather, who has inspired and encouraged all of us to pursue our passions and live our lives to the fullest. He was a Renaissance Man, in the truest sense of the word, and taught me that sometimes, it's ok to take the long and winding path to a goal.

I also dedicate this book to Connor, my brave 10-year-old Type 1 warrior, whose resilience and strength continue to inspire me every day.

To Samantha, Brandon, and Cailyn, Connor's older siblings, I dedicate this book in recognition of your unwavering support and dedication to being caregivers for your brother and for extending your compassion to others with disabilities. You have all made the world a better place just by living with your hearts first.

I also want to thank Jana Hayden, my tireless Editor in Chief, for her invaluable contributions to this project, and to Mark, my loving and supportive husband, for standing by my side through nearly ten years of homework assignments and late-night writing binges.

I'd also like to offer a special thank you to all of the women who contributed to this project. Without their input, this book would never have been possible. Finally, this book is dedicated to all families with children living with diabetes and to those who support them. May this book inspire and empower you in your journey toward better health and well-being.

Contents

Preface

5:22 am. My head shoots off the pillow as I struggle to make sense of my reality. A dream. One of the worst I've had since the diagnosis. Life as the mother of a Type 1 diabetic toddler is rarely easy, but some days—or nights—are worse than others. Tonight I'm suffering from a terrible earache so sleep comes in fitful bursts and Connor's numbers (the way we refer to his blood glucose levels) are worse than usual. In other words, each time my body gives in to fatigue and lets me fall asleep, I'm awoken not too shortly after by the sound of the alarm on his continuous glucose monitor—"Dex".

This time I must have fallen into a deeper sleep than the other times (thanks to the double dose of Extra Strength Tylenol). When the dream wakes me, I check the Dex only to find that he's pretty low—I slept through the last alarm. But my body knew. I dreamt it. Actually, I often dream in numbers. 250—HIGH. 56—LOW. I often find myself waking up frantic just moments before the alarm sounds.

Sometimes it's just that simple. I dream him low or high and wake up. The alarm sounds soon after and I correct with some food or insulin and go back to sleep. But tonight's dream wasn't simple; it was horrifying.

We were being held by terrorists. We were in some type of big conference center with multiple rooms and levels. Connor was LOW and I was desperate to find him a source of carbohydrates before he passed out. I was running, frantically, from room to room begging our captors to let me find him some juice. They did. I returned to find Connor in my husband's firm grasp. Connor was shaking, and his eyes were rolling back in his head. I knew he was about to lose consciousness. I struggled to free the skinny straw from its cellophane sleeve, but the plastic kept breaking apart in little bits between my fingers. I finally loosed the straw from its packaging, but could not get it into the little hole at the top of the juice pouch—each time I tried it bent in resistance. I used my nail to puncture the membrane. I've done this before in real life when the straw has gone missing. Thankfully the trick works in dreams as well.

As I put the straw to his lips and watched his baby Adam's apple bob with each swallow, a sense of calm came over me. "It's going to be ok," I thought. "He's going to be alright." And then I saw it—some type of gas being pushed through the air vents. It didn't matter that I had saved his life just seconds before; I now had to do it all over again.

I sat there in the dark and worked to clear the images of the dream. I knew it would be a while before I could go back to sleep. I have a general rule about avoiding electronics and lights in the middle of the night—I do finger checks by the dim screen light of my phone, and grope the walls when I need to use the bathroom—but occasionally I make exceptions. This night was one of those times.

The exception I make in instances like this is to reach out for support. I turn to Facebook, but not to check my news feed. I go straight to the site that I only wish were a real-live place: Diapers and Diabetes.

At the time I jotted down that terrifying experience, we had been two years into managing this disease—most of that time spent on an island in the middle of the Pacific, far from any type of real support. I had managed to join a number of online support groups, but Diapers and Diabetes was by far my favorite. We're a little old for that group now (at the time of this writing, my son is closing in on 9), and I look more to groups like T1D Mod Squad or Empowering Parents of Children with Celiac Disease and Type 1 Diabetes, but in those early years, D&D was my number one space for support. I still "stop by" every now and again when I feel like I can offer some words of support or wisdom to a parent of a newly diagnosed young one.

Now, when it's 4am and I've been combating lows for three straight hours, I don't usually turn to online support groups for help, but I'm always comforted to know that there's someone out there, ready to listen if I really need some emotional support. We've been at this game for 8 years now, so I generally know what to do when midnight rolls around and the pizza he ate at six is starting to dump carbs into his little body, shooting his numbers higher and higher. But while I might not need suggestions in the heat of the moment, I'm always happy to know that come morning, I can post a screenshot of the rollercoaster glucose readings that I survived the previous night and get a little love from the only ones who truly understand what it's really like to live as the parent of young type 1 diabetic.

The truth is, we all need it. We desperately need that lifeline to keep us going and to remind us that we're not alone in our struggles. And that's why I started writing this book. It took me months to find the D&D group, and longer than that to start building a real network of support. I felt isolated and alone in my struggles and wished every day for a buddy to commiserate with. There were days that I thought my sanity was at grave risk—a problem since I have four children to care for. I sincerely believe that finding others like me, and knowing that my struggles weren't unique gave me the strength I needed to push through that first incredibly trying year. Knowing that dreams like the one I had that fitful night aren't a sign of insanity, but a reflection of the fears we each live with every day, keeps me strong.

The following stories reflect feelings of both strength and weakness; joy and sorrow. I've structured the book that way to help remind everyone out there that while life should be savored, and every child appreciated, the struggles of life as a Type 1 caregiver are real, and weakness is not a crime. I've also woven scientifically-based medical information into each of the stories in the hopes that these sections will serve as resources for parents who need to advocate for themselves and their children in the overwhelming medical community that most parents are unfamiliar with.

When I first started this project, 7 years ago, I only envisioned interviewing other mothers. The planned book was an offshoot of an article I had written to help support women, like myself, who were still nursing their child at the time of diagnosis. The common practice was (and still often is) to discourage nursing mothers from breastfeeding because there is a fear that breastmilk is too difficult to calculate and therefore overly complicates an already difficult practice. I've worked hard to dispel that myth (both in my original article and in some of the stories that follow). But I also realized that there was a bigger story that needed to be told. As a result, this book has taken on several new forms, as I've come to recognize how powerful the complex support network is for each young diabetic.

There will likely be a different feel to the stories that were written earlier in the project than those that came later. Some of this difference is a reflection of some of my own evolution over the years, but I think there is also a unique distinction between the experience of a mother nearly losing a child, to that of other caregivers who come into the fold over time. In the original stories told by the mothers, each one in turn told me of the different triggers that bring her back to that single moment in time when everything changed. For one it's the sight of an ambulance racing by with its sirens blaring. For another, it's the trip down a random tree-lined back road that reminds her of the route to the hospital. Whatever it is that brings each woman back, she will revisit that moment all too frequently—possibly with even more clarity than the day she gave birth and first became a mother.

For some women, especially those who have been managing their child's illness for several years, there is a complexity to their story well beyond the day of diagnosis. Those narratives have been broken up throughout the book, with different aspects of their experiences appearing according to chapter subjects. My experiences with Connor, on the other hand, follow below as one continuous narrative, covering everything from our early days in the hospital, to more recent events, such as his celiac diagnosis.

I hope you'll enjoy the stories of these families who have generously shared both their time and experiences to make this book a reality. ~Erin~

Chapter One

Young Diabetics through the Years

"I have taken insulin for 82 years—never missed a shot." These are the words of 90-year-old Gladys Dull during a 2007 interview with Chana Joffe-Walt for PRX. At the time of this interview, Gladys was the oldest living individual with Type 1 diabetes.

"When I was just 7 years old—I wasn't quite 7—I vomited and had to go to the bathroom all the time," She recalls with a slight chuckle that hints at her embarrassment. "We didn't know anybody with diabetes. Well, they got me on the insulin, and I got along fine—that was in 1924."

The way Gladys describes those early days, one might think the use of insulin was as commonplace as it is today. At the time of her diagnosis, Gladys had just lost her parents to the Great Influenza (or Spanish Flu) and was growing up with family in North Dakota —an area of the country that would soon become synonymous with the American Dustbowl. She was a long way from the bustling cities of the East Coast, and even further from Toronto, Canada, where Frederick Banting and his team were desperately trying to hand-fill bottles of insulin made from ground-up, distilled, animal pancreas.

After a brief period of illness, children today—at least in America—are usually diagnosed fairly quickly, put on insulin, and get along just fine. What Gladys' words don't convey is that her 1924 diagnosis couldn't have been better timed. From the time Fredrick Banting and his colleague Charles Best had officially discovered insulin roughly four years earlier, it would take another three years for a successful method of mass production to be developed. For the majority of people diagnosed in the early twenties, a diagnosis of diabetes still carried with it a prognosis of certain death. While Banting and his team had managed to move on from the original process of using dog pancreas to that of beef and pork (mainly because they were running out of dogs), turning the ground tissue into a purified clear liquid that could be injected into the human body was no simple process. Banting and his team had moved on to grinding up the beef and pork tissue in large machines—much as a meat factory would do to make sausage—resulting in pancreatic extracts that were relatively impure. The house physician at Toronto General Hospital described what he injected into the buttocks of 14-year-old Leonard Thompson as "15 cc of thick brown muck."

Despite the fact that Banting and Best still had work to do on refining their product, the feedback from early trials was impressive. In The Discovery of Insulin, Michael Bliss describes the impact that the discovery of insulin in the winter of 1921-22 had on the diabetic community:

"Those who watched the first starved, sometimes comatose, diabetics receive insulin and return to life saw one of the genuine miracles of modern medicine. They were present at the closest approach to the resurrection of the body that our secular society can achieve, and at the discovery of what has become the elixir of life for millions of human beings around the world."

Bliss's words are powerful. The clear liquid that fills little glass vials, and is measured in fractions of a milliliter, truly is an elixir of life for my son and millions of other diabetics. We guard those precious vials with our lives—or at least insulated sleeves within padded pockets of further insulated carrying cases. I'm sure I've walked around with less care for gold on my wrist or money in my pocket than I do for my son's insulin. But to truly appreciate the value of this watery substance, we have to go back to a time before it existed.

What I learned somewhat recently is that the concept of diabetes—the recognition of a disease that causes the body to evacuate fluids at an unnaturally high rate, and that somehow relates to sugar levels in urine—has been around since the ancient Egyptians. Robert Tattersall goes into great depth about the evolution of diabetes research in his book Diabetes: The Biography from its first recording on Egyptian papyrus in 1500 BCE, through the Dark Ages (which truly were dark in terms of medical science!) and the evolution of medical technology through the twentieth century. It's a bit more comprehensive than anything I could cover here, but I do believe a brief overview of the evolutionary process can be helpful when trying to gain some perspective on how having a child with Type 1 diabetes impacts quality of life—and how much worse off we would all be if living just even a century ago.

For thousands of years doctors recognized that individuals who exhibited the symptoms of diabetes also had sugar in their urine. They knew this because they frequently tasted urine (and other bodily substances) as a means of diagnosing diseases. According to James Bradley of the Washington Post, "The history of diagnosis has been the history of doctors' use of the five senses." In a better effort to understand bodily processes and the characteristics of various conditions, sampling blood, urine, and even semen was just part of the job-description.

While their dedication to the practice of healing is admirable, it's quite obvious that such a system of analysis doesn't lead to highly accurate data collection or disease management. "This urine tastes sweeter than that urine" doesn't really yield the type of information one needs to accurately keep blood glucose levels in check. But it was a start. Throughout the 1700 and 1800s, doctors continued to investigate the correlation between diabetic symptoms and sweetened urine but were entirely uncertain as to the cause of the phenomenon.

One of the most interesting discoveries came in 1780 when doctors learned that much like grapes or apples, diabetic urine could be fermented. Within three days of mixing yeast with 24 pints of a diabetic patient's urine, Dr. Francis Home found that a "tolerable" beer was born. Three cheers for medical science!

Over the years, many doctors assumed a connection between food and diabetes, and a whole host of diets have been prescribed—from those emphasizing the need for restriction to protein and/or fat-based diets, to others allowing for low-starch carbohydrates like almonds, or even high-sugar diets designed to replace the sugars lost through urination. Some experts proclaimed that certain foods (such as oats, legumes, lime water, or rancid meats) were sure to cure the disease altogether. Much of this still goes on today with "naturalists" claiming to have discovered a sure-fire way to cure diabetes without ever having to take medicine again. While such antics might have been understandable in the late 19th century, such empty promises spark bitter debates across social media platforms today.

Of all the dietary protocols prescribed throughout the years, it seems none were as restrictive or potentially life-threatening as the infamous Dr. Allen starvation diet. The doctor himself acknowledged that some patients would die of starvation before succumbing to the actual disease. On a basic level, Dr. Allen was viewed as something of a doctor of death, and parents considered a visit with him a very last resort. At a time when medical experts fully understood the capacity for damage that carbohydrates (and to lesser extent, but still significant, fats and proteins) had on the diabetic body, Dr. Allen offered hope for prolonged life by restricting patients to roughly 400 calories per day. Many would say that reducing an individual to so few calories amounted to little more than torture and that such a life was barely living at all, but at a time when the medical community seemed on the brink of a major discovery, many patients and their families chose a miserable but prolonged life over surely sudden death.

By the time it was over, the Spanish flu would claim fifty million lives worldwide, more than three times the number killed in World War I...But even the flu had a more optimistic prognosis than juvenile diabetes. While the mortality rate for the influenza of 1918 was between 2 and 20 percent, the mortality rate for juvenile diabetes was very nearly 100 percent.

And so Dr. Allen's prescription for starvation endured. One of the doctor's first patients, and one who lived to endure the radical treatment longest, was Elizabeth Hughes, daughter of Charles Evan Hughes, whose political career carried him from the Governor's office of New York state to the United States Supreme Court, and eventually on to a bid for the presidency—a campaign that was lost to Democrat Woodrow Wilson, who at the time seemed the more likely candidate to keep Americans out of the Great War.

By the time Elizabeth was diagnosed and Dr. Allen's radical program had taken root in the spring of 1919, America had not only joined the war, but spent over $30 billion dollars on the war effort and sacrificed the lives of over 100,000 to battle and disease. This expenditure of money, resources, and lives naturally diverted attention from diabetes research, but as the war came to a close and doctors returned home, renewed interest in finding a cure would quickly prove successful.

One doctor—an Army surgeon by the name of Fredrick Banting—would prove instrumental in the discovery of insulin in the years immediately following the war. As the story goes (and there are plenty floating around about this man who is considered a savior by millions of diabetics worldwide) Banting was forced to take on some lecturing hours at the local university as he tried to make ends meet while building up his medical practice in his new hometown of London, Canada. In preparation for a lecture on the pancreas—one he was dreading due to his poor knowledge on the subject matter—he spent some hours reading through published articles on the topic. After a restless night of sleep, he awoke at 2 am to an epiphany—an idea for how the "diabetes hormone" could be extracted from a dog's pancreas and used to supplement the hormone deficiency in individuals whose pancreas was no longer functioning properly.

"Oct 31/20. Diabetus." Banting's note begins. "Ligate (tie off) pancreatic ducts of dog. Keep dogs alive till acini degenerate leaving islets. Try to isolate the internal secretion of these to relieve glycosuria (sugar in the urine)."

What Banting didn't know at the time was that there had been multiple failed attempts over the years to obtain and utilize canine pancreatic extract and there had even been direct studies using such a serum to treat animals who had artificially been put in a diabetic state for the purpose of research. Even Banting himself would come to say that it was better he hadn't known the odds were stacked against him as such knowledge might have kept him from pressing forward.

When Banting approached Professor Macleod, a senior professor at the university, about borrowing lab space to experiment on dogs to test his theory, Macleod was unimpressed with Banting's lack of knowledge on the subject and wrote in his notes, "I found that Dr. Banting had only a superficial textbook knowledge of the work that had been done and no familiarity with the methods by which such a problem could be investigated in the laboratory." Despite his lack of faith in Banting, Macleod agreed to give Banting use of the lab and two students for assistance to be used on a rotating basis. Charles Best, winning a coin toss to determine who would assist first, went on to become Banting's partner for the next several months, and it would actually be Best who would deliver the first medical dose of insulin to a human patient on January 11, 1922.

The early days of success, however were quickly overshadowed by the realization that the production of insulin in any sufficient quantity could not be accomplished in a college lab room. As Jim Turner explains in his three-part special Novo Story of Insulin, "the Toronto team was overwhelmed. They needed more money. Better facilities. And most importantly, time to figure out the complex chemical work [of turning ground-up pancreas into purified insulin]. But time was not something they had on their side."

The research team spent countless hours playing with measurements and working to distill the concoctions using old-school beakers and single burners, just to produce small batches of the life-saving hormone. Without a means of mass-production, there would be no way for doctors to meet the demands of the diabetic population. As Turner goes on to say, "There seemed an insurmountable gap between healing a single patient and mass-producing the miracle hormone."

All of that would change in late 1923 when both George Clowes of Eli Lilly in Indianapolis and Dr. August Krogh of Denmark independently approached Banting and his team with requests to start applying methods of mass production to Banting and Best's process. Reluctantly the Canadian team agreed to both requests. George Clowes—driven by a sense for business—and Dr. Krogh—driven by the desire to save his own wife who had been recently diagnosed—soon began mass production on two continents. Krogh went on to found Novo Nordisk, and with Clowes heading Research and Development for Eli Lilly, two of the world's leading drug manufacturers were born. The future of diabetes management was officially changed forever.

For patients like Gladys Dull, and Elizabeth Hughes, the new innovations in insulin distribution came just in time. Millions of people's lives around the world that would have been lost just the year before were spared as a result of the commercialization of insulin. Bob Cleveland and his brother Gerald were another two such fortunate benefactors of the revised production process. But as they explain, diabetes management was still much more crude than it is today. There were no finely tuned long-lasting and fast-acting insulins that could be used to carefully regulate blood sugar throughout the day. Successful control still depended on careful adherence to a prescribed diet. Patients were told exactly how many grams of carbohydrates they could take in each day and were directed to take two to three shots daily to counteract the intake.

"I remember my mother said I was skin and bones when I did go to the hospital," Bob explains. "Occasionally, she'd have to buy a loaf of sliced bread. A slice of that bread would be maybe thirty grams, so she'd have to cut a piece of it off or cut the crust off so that I only had twenty grams."

Bob's brother, Gerald, who was diagnosed a few years later, says, "When I was diagnosed, I felt that the world kind of dumped in on me, and I was going to have a different kind of life."

And while many diabetic patients and their families suggest the same concern today—that life drastically changes with a diabetes diagnosis, Gerald reminds us of how painfully different it was back then: "We had needles that had to be sharpened with a wet stone and boiled up after every use."

There weren't disposable syringes like there are now, and the tools for monitoring blood sugar were nowhere near as precise or easy to manage. As Jim Turner explains, "There were no quick blood tests or easy home kits. Readings required boiling urine samples in a test tube with chemicals multiple times each day."

Diabetes was no longer a death sentence, but life was not easy either. Both of the Cleveland brothers talk about their efforts to keep their disease a secret from everyone outside of their immediate family. In talking about the early days of dating his wife, Bob says, "We dated for about six months before she found out that I was a diabetic. I was afraid she would back off just like employers did when they found out."

Over the next several decades, little would change in the world of diabetes management. The 1950s saw a series of innovations in what would become the birth of the computer era, and In July of 1969, Edwin Aldrin (Buzz) and Neil Armstrong would be the first individuals to set foot on the moon. On April 3, 1973 the first cellular phone call was made, and in 1978 England celebrated the birth of the world's first test-tube baby. But there just didn't seem to be much change in the field of diabetes research.

As Michael Bliss explains, there "really [were] no breakthroughs in insulin production—very frustrating for everybody—until in the early 1980s you entered a new era." For the first time in roughly sixty years, scientists were able to use DNA science to replicate human insulin genes, which meant an end to the extraction of pancreatic serum from animals. Not only was this a huge relief for people worried about the potential risks of using animal extracts for medicine, it also meant an end to supply worries. The new DNA-based process also meant the ability to produce more advanced forms of insulin with distinct long-lasting and fast-acting products that would lead to more precise glucose control. And of course, disposable syringes, portable home glucose monitors that can read small droplets of blood, and electronic delivery and monitoring systems like insulin pumps and continuous glucose monitors (CGMs) continue to revolutionize the way people manage this disease.

Despite the innovations, some people like Gladys stuck with the old ways, mixing urine with Benedict's solution and boiling it to check for blood sugars or working with glass syringes. In the later years, after Gladys had outlived her husband and was being cared for by her son Norm, the doctor was surprised to find that she was still doing things the old-fashioned way. When the doctor asked about Gladys' blood sugar, Norm replied, "Grayish-brick." As Norm recalls, "He couldn't understand what I was talking about. He couldn't believe that she had never taken a blood test."

Fortunately, the newest generation of Type 1 kids will never have to know the struggles of the young heroes and heroines who survived the starvation diets and imprecise doses of muddy insulin. While there is still no cure for diabetes, and much of the most recent technology (from pumps and CGMs to the more advanced "artificial pancreas" or islet cell transplant therapy) is still well outside the reach of the average patient, we are all still a lot better off than those in our not-so-distant past.

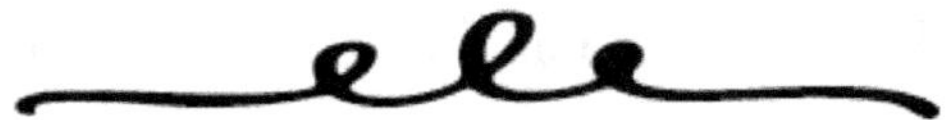

Footnotes For Chapter 1:

Joffe-Walt, Chana. "90-Year Old is a Living History of Diabetes." PRX. The Public Radio Exchange, 1 Jan. 2007. Web. 25 Mar. 2016. Hirsch, James. "The Durable Diabetic: Gladys Dull Relies on the Basics to Make Medical History." DiaTribe. The DiaTribe Foundation, 07 June 2007. Web. 25 Mar. 2016. Tattersall, 57 This characteristic actually applies specifically to diabetes mellitus (aptly named in reference to the Latin word for honey). Diabetes insipidus would come to be distinguished as a separate relative of the disease—characterized by similar outward symptoms such as frequent thirst and urination, but unique in that the urine lacked the sweetness of diabetes mellitus patients (Bliss, 20). From Tattersall's Diabetes: The Biography (15). "One diet that had a short vogue in the 1850s was sugar feeding, brainchild of the well-known but eccentric French physician Pierre Piorry (1794-1879). He thought that diabetics lost weight and felt so weak because of the amount of sugar they lost in the urine and that replacing it should restore strength" (Tattersall, 20). Cooper and Ainsberg, 26. Cooper and Ainsberg, 21. Cooper and Ainsberg, 17. This note is now part of the archives at the Academy of Medicine in Toronto, and countless images of it are found in books and online regarding it as the official turning point in the war against diabetes. Breecher, and Anderson In the end Banting and Macleod would be named as the recipients of the Nobel Prize for their discovery of insulin. This was a subject of discontent for Banting who believed that Best was more instrumental in the research and ultimate success of refining insulin for human use. Tattersall, 54-57. Turner, Jim. "Novo Story of Insulin." DLife. 1 Feb. 2010. YouTube. Web. 25 Mar. 2016. The Cleveland's brother's words are documented as part of Jim Turner's documentary "Novo Story of Insulin—Part 3." Seward, "The First Mobile Phone Call" "90th Anniversary Issue: 1970s" This quote comes from his commentary in Part 3 of Turner's documentary, not Bliss' book. Turner, Part 3 More information on these developments can be found at the National Institute of Diabetes and Digestive and Kidney Diseases and Diabetes Forecast: The Healthy Living Magazine.

CHAPTER TWO

Our Story

This chapter serves as a glimpse into the early days of my son Connor's diagnosis. Connor's story will be told from both my perspective and that of my mother. The rest of the book is filled with other families' stories, collected through oral interviews, social media posts, and emails. These tales serve as a reminder of the profound responsibility that comes with caring for a loved one with an invisible disease, especially when the caregiver does not have a medical background.

While there are plenty of events—both good and bad—that have colored my experiences over the past several years since Connor was first hospitalized, the essence of my life as a mother of a special needs child all filters back to that single moment in time when he was diagnosed. And so that's where my story will begin. ~Erin~

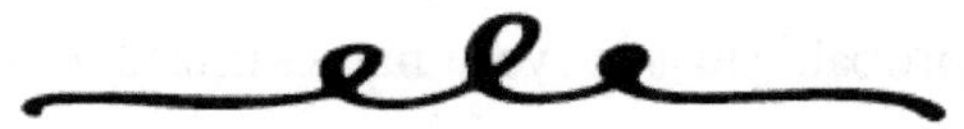

Erin & Connor

As the months have faded into years, I've often found myself reflecting on the fact that while certain details of the defining moments in a person's life can be so vivid, others can be so blank. Some specifics won't come back no matter how hard I try to recall them, yet there are others I'll never forget regardless of how badly I wish I could. For example, I still remember watching my husband—Mark—slide down the wall and crash to the floor as the doctor gave the diagnosis. "Diabetes". The diagnosis wasn't for him of course, but as any parent will attest, it may as well have been. Connor was only 15 months old at the time making the blow that much harder to handle.

Type One comes from my side, or so I think. There is some debate regarding the genetic nature of Type 1 diabetes, but I'll leave that discussion for another writing project. Either way, as if my young son's diagnosis wasn't enough in itself, my forty-seven year old cousin—the only one I had known to that point with type-one diabetes—had just died a few weeks earlier from disease-related complications. I had just seen her a few months earlier (after not having seen her for years) at a family reunion. She came up to me at one point in that evening, annoyed at the fact that some more distant relative had just addressed her, apparently quite certain of themselves, as if she was the oldest of her sisters.

"Can you believe he thought I was the oldest?"

"I'm sure he wasn't trying to say that you looked the oldest," I tried to console her. "He probably just got your names mixed up. This is such a big family—when I was younger I always used to get your names confused!"

To be honest, I wasn't exactly sure that the mix-up had simply been a flip-flop of names. When I initially saw her, I thought she looked quite a bit older to me than I had remembered from the last time I had seen her. She was the youngest in the family, but it seemed to me then, that the years of battling this terrible disease had left her looking older than she really was. In talking to one of her sisters after the fact, I learned that others didn't share my perceptions, but my initial shock upon seeing her was what I wrestled with during those first hours in the hospital.

As I stood there processing the doctor's words about my son, the interaction of that night flashed before me. Was this my baby's destiny?

I was brought back from the reverie by Mark's crying. I remember listening to—but at the same time not really hearing—his conversations on the phone. First with his mom. Then his step-dad Mike, the cardiologist. At that point, any direct connection to the medical community seemed like a lifeline. And anything that kept him out of the room where Connor was, was a blessing.

"It's good he has someone to talk to" the nurse said of my husband in a brief moment of calm. "I don't really think it's good for him to be in here." And she was right. Every time he looked at Connor—the seemingly lifeless body strapped with tubes and wires—he became hysterical. For whatever reason, I wasn't. I just went into crisis-management mode. My then 4 year-old daughter Cailyn, who had been carted off with us because we had no one to leave her with, sat shell-shocked in a chair in the corner of the room. She didn't cry. She just stared, wide-eyed, at all the craziness going on around her. I bounced back and forth between her and Connor, alternately whispering into each of their ears.

"It's ok sweetie. He's going to be ok. The doctors are taking good care of him."Quickly followed by a scurry to the bed and a whisper into the unresponsive ear, "It's ok baby. Mommy's here. The doctors are taking good care of you. You're going to be ok."

In some ways, those hushed conversations were my rock. I had a purpose—to keep my babies from sensing fear—and nothing else mattered.

Periodically I'd ask irrationally calm questions of the nurses. "You still can't get the IV line," I remarked to the one. "Is there another option if his veins are too compromised?" Where did these words come from? I knew what was happening. He was in such a severe state of dehydration that his veins had collapsed and the nurses couldn't get even the tiniest needle into any of them. But somehow I remained calm.

I don't remember if I thought it at the moment, or if it was something that occurred to me afterward, but I knew my own mother would be proud. She was always there for me and my brother in times of emergency—no matter how ugly things got. She had held my hand and calmed my fears when I was twelve and the doctor who was about to shove a two-inch needle into my Achilles told me, "Here, put this pillow on your face. I have other patients." And she had been there for me four years later when the doctor had to draw fluid from my kneecap after a skiing accident where I tore my meniscus. And like her, here I was for my own children making sure that both kids knew that as long as mommy was there, everything would be ok. And so I remained calm.

Everything leading up to us sitting in that room had happened in a state of chaos—from the blizzard swirling outside, to the mad-dash to get the older ones shuffled off to various neighbors two hours before the school bus was due to arrive. We had gone to sleep the night before thinking that Connor had caught his older brother's stomach bug. But when I woke in those early morning hours, bathed in his urine, which had also soaked our sheets, I looked at his face, and knew something much worse than the flu was going on. In those pre-dawn shadows, I could just barely make out his features, but I sensed an eeriness to his face. His eyes were sunken, almost alien-like. It was the spookiest look I had ever seen.

I was actually scheduled to bring him to the doctor that morning for a well-visit and his first shots. I had originally planned to start him with vaccines when he turned one, but he was too sick at that scheduled visit and the doctor and I agreed it would be best to hold off. That was September. We rescheduled for October, but he was sick again. Actually, he seemed to be getting sick a lot at that point, but with three older siblings and it being the start of cold and flu season, we just brushed off the recurring sicknesses as normal. And so there we found ourselves in December, ready for the much anticipated well-visit, only to find him sick again. Only this time there wouldn't be a postponement. Actually, as we looked at his face, we knew that we couldn't wait even another hour to see the doctor. I called her and explained his symptoms. The office wasn't even open yet, but she told us she'd meet us there in twenty minutes.

We called around to each of the neighbors until we found someone who could take the two oldest ones to feed them breakfast and get them off to school. It was so incredibly cold—December in Chicago—but we didn't want to take the time to warm up the car so we bundled up the two little ones—Connor and his 4-year-old sister Cailyn—and rushed off.

Fortunately, the doctor's office was just down the road. On nice days I had even walked there with the kids. Mark squeaked into the parking lot and urged us out. "I'll bring KK"—our nickname for the 4-year-old—"once I park the car. You two just go."

I walked through the front door and by the look on the doctor's face, knew the situation wasn't good. I think Mark knew all along that we wouldn't be staying. He left the car running right outside and poked his head in to see what the plan was.

"It's not good," the doctor told us. "This is not the flu. You need to get him to the hospital right away." On those words, Mark ran right back out the door.

"Is he ok to drive?" She asked me in response to the crazed look that we had both seen on his face. "Yeah, he'll be fine", I assured her, and she gave me a hug. "Hurry."

When we arrived at the hospital there was a line, but the intake nurse took one look at Connor and knew that he couldn't wait. She rushed us into private room and called for help. There was an instant flurry of activity and he was quickly carted off to an emergency room. The doctors and nurses were too preoccupied with trying to stabilize his little body to talk to us, but eventually we would learn that they had confirmed their initial suspicions of Type 1 diabetes and that his glucose level was over 850; he was in a severe state of DKA; his veins had collapsed and he was unconscious.

"We're still not sure how much damage has been done," one doctor told me. "We'll have to do some tests and check for brain damage, but first we have to stabilize him." In that moment, everything just seemed to slow down.

The head nurse eventually made the decision to tap the jugular vein in his neck—there are no words that can touch what I felt at that moment.

"I'll probably get in trouble for doing that," she said to me. "But if it had been my grandson, I would have done the same thing. You have a very sick little boy. I was just trying to save his life."

"I understand. I'm glad someone was finally able to get an IV," I reassured her. Still today, when he gets angry or upset, his vein bulges in that place where the catheter was inserted—an all-too vivid transportation back to that day.

It took hours for the ambulance to arrive for our transport to the children's hospital. In the meantime, we endured one procedure after the next. At some point, Mark's mother came to pick up Cailyn. I can't remember a word that was spoken between the two of us—just the tears and heartbreak in her eyes. Honestly, I couldn't look at her for long because her face reflected every emotion I was desperately struggling to hold back. I was just grateful that my four-year-old didn't have to sit in a corner anymore, watching the horror unfold around her. I was relieved that I could take a break from splitting myself trying to reassure her, while also trying to tend to Connor.

At some point, someone told me, "If you had waited a few more hours to bring him in, he'd be dead."

Not soon after, I watched as they pushed Connor's gurney into the MRI tunnel so they could check for brain damage. I like to think of him as still unconscious in that moment—as if none of this was bothering him—but when I look at the photos I took that day, I'm reminded that he wasn't. The IV was working, and as the life-saving fluid filled his veins, he awoke to a nightmare. He started screaming. With straps on his arms, legs, and across his forehead, he was completely immobilized. The only things that could move were his eyes and his mouth. And as he screamed, he looked at me with sheer terror. And there was nothing I could do.

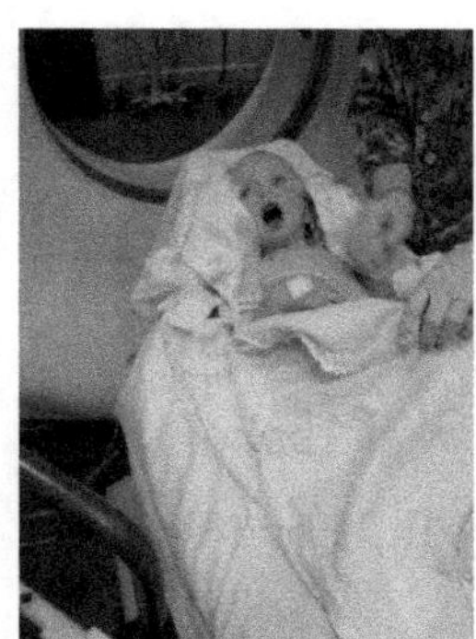
Connor being wheeled into the MRI machine

Eventually, we were carted back to the triage room to wait for the ambulance. Someone brought me a breast pump because I wasn't allowed to nurse him and we had already skipped two feedings. Most toddlers wouldn't be nursing that frequently at his age—actually, in this country, most toddlers don't nurse at all—but he still was. Actually, he had been refusing most solid foods for months, and was becoming more and more dependent on my milk. I had attributed it to teething and the various sicknesses he had been fighting off. In hindsight, I've often wondered if his little body knew that as his pancreas shut down, it couldn't handle the more complex carbohydrates found in table food. Of course, that's not based on any kind of science—just mommy speculation.

Eventually, the ambulance arrived. I can't for the life of me remember what the lead EMT looked like, or what she was wearing, but I do remember the look of horror on her face when she saw the IV coming out of his neck.

"Why is there an IV in his neck?" she exclaimed. I explained how difficult it had been for them to find a vein that could hold the IV.

"I've got a trick for that," she said. She shut off the lights in the room and came back to the bed. She lifted his little hand and put a flashlight up to his palm. All of his tiny little veins shone blue beneath his pale skin.

"See. This one will work just fine." And she inserted a catheter, securing it off so that the IV could be transitioned to his hand. In the hospital nurse's defense, Connor had already been given several bags of IV fluids by this time, so it's likely his veins were simply plumping up again, but at that moment, the EMT's air of confidence gave me a fresh sense of hope. I knew things were going to be ok.

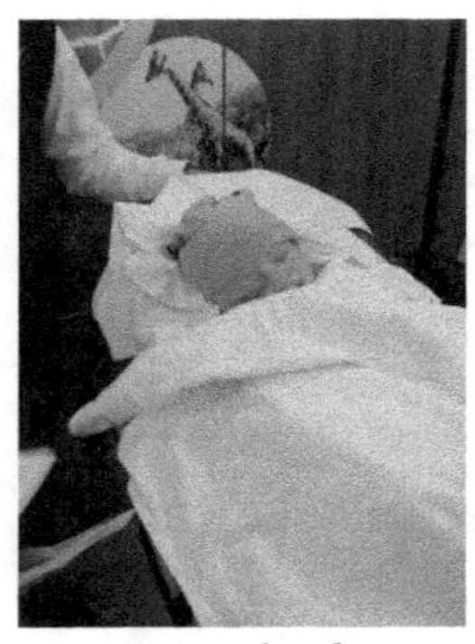

Connor in his little froggie hat that the EMT gave him for the transfer to the children's hospital

One of the ambulance crew members had a little froggie hat with him and put it on Connor's head so he wouldn't be cold when we transitioned from the hospital to the ambulance. With that oversized bright green hat on his head, his little body seemed to shrink a little more.

As they helped me into the ambulance, Mark went to retrieve the car so that he could gather our things from home and make longer-term arrangements for the other kids. As we pulled away from the loading station, I told the EMT what the one nurse had said to me—that they had never seen a case so bad, and that he was lucky to be alive; that in a matter of just a few more hours he would surely have been dead. I remember her reassuring words: "I've seen much worse. And they've survived—without complications." I don't know if I thanked her in that moment, but I will be forever grateful for her reassuring words.

As she explained to me, it is incredibly rare to see an older person present with diabetes for the first time with numbers so high, but it is quite common in little ones. They can't talk. They can't tell you that they're not feeling well, and that something is really off. For the ER workers, who mostly work with adults, I guess this really was the worst case they had ever seen. For a Children's Hospital EMT, who works with young children and infants every day, this unfortunately wasn't.

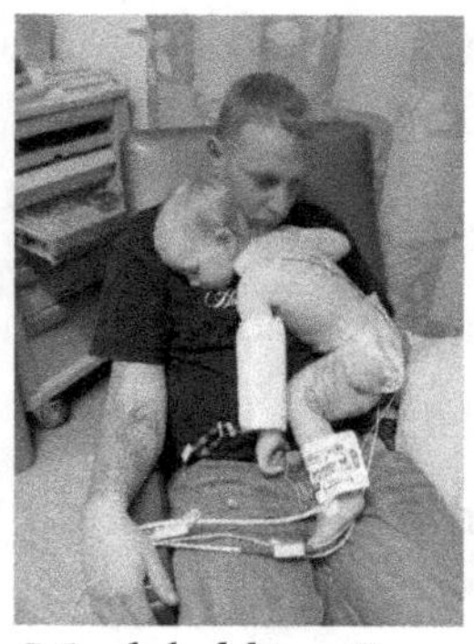
Mark holding Connor in the very early days--wires still attached

Daddy's heart was absolutely breaking in those first hours.

Other than her reassurances that everything would be ok, I can't recall anything of that ambulance ride, even though it lasted over an hour. At this point, memory seems to come in flashes—like from a dream. I feel like there was some type of revolving floor that allowed the ambulance to turn around in a confined space. But I'm not sure if that is a real memory or something I had just seen somewhere before. Maybe in a movie. I remember something of an elevator. Vaguely. Like there's a memory trying to push through—the music, the lights, the kid-friendly characters painted on the walls. But maybe that was from later in the week from the countless trips I made up and down to the hospital cafeteria.

While I can't clearly picture the transition to our room in the PIKU, I do remember desperately wanting to nurse my son. Nursing was still a big part of not only his nutrition, but his comfort and I wasn't allowed to give him either. The best I could do was bend down into the plastic crib and put my cheek to his cheek. And cry. I remember such a swirl of emotions. Anger at the nurses for denying me the ability to care for my son the only way I knew how, and frustration with myself for not knowing how to mother him any other way.

"We can still give you the breastfeeding mom coupons," someone told me—as if credit for free food in the cafeteria was some type of consolation prize. Eventually, determination set in. I had just recently received my IBCLC certification and belonged to a number of professional groups geared toward supporting nursing mothers. I was sure someone would have information to help me prove that breastfeeding my son was safe. Unfortunately, I was wrong. I reached out to countless friends and colleagues, but no one had anything to offer.

"There just doesn't seem to be any research on breastfeeding a diabetic child," I was told over and over again. But I knew enough about breastfeeding management to feel confident that the carbohydrates in breastmilk could be calculated (or at least estimated) just like any other food, and I challenged the nurses to give me medical reasons why breastmilk couldn't be factored into his plan just like anything else.

"We just don't know how to calculate his intake," they explained. "How can we know how much he's getting and how much insulin he needs to cover it?"

"I'll look it up," I assured them. "I know that there are tables with nutritional facts for breastmilk."

"That won't be good enough," one told me. "If it's information that comes from outside of this hospital, we can't accept it. We need something that comes from hospital guidelines... He's over a year old anyway. It's not like he needs it anymore."

I couldn't believe the ridiculous words I was hearing. What they were telling me was that no matter what scientific evidence I came back with, it just wouldn't be good enough—because as far as they were concerned, it just wasn't worth it. I really started to think that all hope was lost.

And then we had our miracle. A nutritionist from the endocrinology team came to see me. "I heard that you want to breastfeed your son and that they're giving you a hard time," she said to me.

I couldn't believe it. It seemed like this woman was actually there to advocate for me. "I understand. I nursed my own kids into toddlerhood and I know how important it is," she explained. "Eventually we'll have to get a rough estimate of how much you produce by seeing what you pump, but for now, put him to your breast. He needs that comfort more than anything—and so do you."

And so I cried. "Thank you."

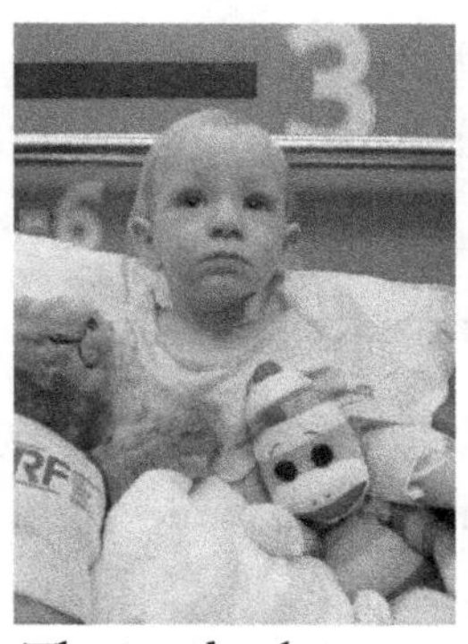

The insulin has started working! Five days after diagnosis and tubes are out; it's time for a wagon ride.

We survived those first twenty-four hours and the week that followed; sharing a little room, crowded with wires, dirty clothes, and the clichéd but appropriate tension you could cut with a knife. At one point they almost threw my husband out because the two of us could not stop fighting over every little thing. They thought maybe it would be best to separate us. "We're fine. We'll control ourselves," we promised.

While we did our best to control our emotions, the tension built every hour that we came closer to release. My husband wasn't sure that we were ready to care for him on our own. I couldn't stand another minute looking at those walls. And then there was the other issue: We had a shipping container arriving at our house in two days and we were scheduled to depart for Maui (a return to our previous home) in less than two weeks.

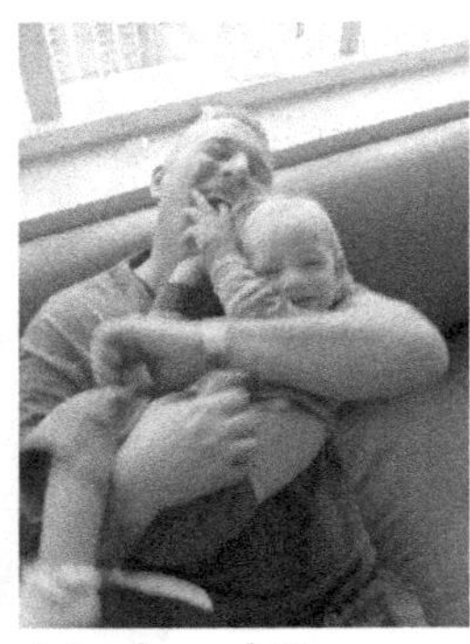

Mark and Connor sharing some laughs for the first time since diagnosis

Everything was about to change dramatically. Connor had been diagnosed on Friday, the 13th of December. We didn't leave the hospital until the 18th, and the shipping container was scheduled to be picked up on the 21st. I had plane tickets for myself and the kids with a departure date of December 31st. Mark was scheduled to work two weeks into January and meet up with us at the end of that month, and my mom had her ticket to accompany me and the kids since my new job was scheduled to start on January 6th—the first day of the new semester at Iao Intermediate school.

The move was certainly change enough (though gratefully we were simply returning to our home on Maui rather than just starting fresh somewhere new); the bigger shift would result from our change in family dynamic. Whereas I had been the stay-at-home parent since Connor was born, Mark and I were about to switch roles. I was going back to full-time teaching, and we agreed that Mark would stay home for a while with Connor and Cailyn until we found the right day-care solution for them, and he found a feasible job opportunity. To say that Mark was terrified at the prospect of caring for Connor on his own would be a major understatement. Not only were we both new to managing Connor's care, Connor was still nursing (thanks to that wonderful nutritionist) and not taking a bottle.

And so Mark stalled. "Maybe we shouldn't go," he said. We can call off the container and cancel the plane tickets."

"But I have a job starting in two weeks. And you already quit yours," I reasoned.

"They'll take me back. They need the help."

"But you're miserable here. You're working fifty hours a week and for what? We can barely put food on the table," I reminded him. "You leave in the pitch dark and come home dog tired in more dark. This is not a life for you. It's not a life for any of us."

"You're sure about this?" He asked.

"I'm sure. You know this is what we have to do."

And so we pushed forward with the plans. His aunts came each day to help us pack and throw out the things we wouldn't take with us. We lived through each day of the following few weeks as a series of sleep-deprived motions interwoven with tearful goodbyes. Mark's bosses gave him the remainder of the year off as paid leave, so he never actually had to return to work at all, and he rescheduled his flight so that he could meet up with us a few days after we settled in. My mom went back home soon after he arrived on island, with plans to come back and visit with my dad in the summer.

We made it through those early months back on Maui the best we could—with six of us crammed into a small two-bedroom apartment, packed with all of the furniture we had taken with us from our former three-level house. We had difficulty keeping Connor in range; Mark was stressed beyond belief and desperate to get back to work, and we often found ourselves wondering if we'd actually be able to survive our new reality.

In June of that year, my parents came back for a visit and helped us buy a house. Money was tight because Mark was only working part-time, and I was only getting a partial summer salary because I had only taught half the year. We had new stresses for sure, but the larger living accommodations gave us all a bit more breathing room. We found a wonderful day-care center that was willing to take Connor on a trial basis. We started him out part-time at the end of the school year and throughout the summer so that he could get used to being there, and the teachers could get used to managing his care before I had to go back to full-time work. The staff members were incredibly caring, but they weren't trained medical professionals. They wouldn't use needles, and when equipment failed (as it often did), they couldn't change it. There were many days where his blood sugar skyrocketed to over 500 or crashed under forty—sometimes more than once in a single day.

The school I had started with when we landed on island was 30 minutes away from our home and his school. When a problem arose, it meant I had to leave work for the day. Fortunately, I managed to get a job for the new school year back at the school I had worked at before leaving the island two years earlier. It was less than two miles from Connor's day care center. We were now almost a year into our new lives, feeling more at ease with our ability to care for him, and more relaxed knowing that I would be close should problems arise.

For the time being, things seemed to settle down. I taught that school year with relatively little drama, though I often had to take emergency calls in class and occasionally had to find coverage so that I could run to address a medical problem. My parents sold their house in New York and bought a place just a mile from where we lived so that they could help us out more. Things weren't easy, but they were manageable.

And then came summer. Mark took Connor back to Chicago to visit family. He struggled to keep Connor's numbers in range—partly because he was unaccustomed to caring for Connor on his own at this point—but also because there seemed to be other medical issues at play. Unfortunately, it would take us four months to figure out exactly what was going on.

"Erin—Wake up!" He yelled into the phone at me one night. It was 3 am and I was actually deep asleep for the first time in ages—not having to manage Connor's nighttime care. They had been away for almost two weeks, and it was almost time for them to take the return flight back home.

"Wake up, I need you!"

"What's going on?" I asked in a fairly irritated voice. This was not the first time since they had left that he called me at some ridiculous time of the morning only because it was daylight in Chicago.

"We're on our way to the hospital." He explained. "Connor crashed and I didn't know what to do so I gave him glucagon ."

"What? Why did you do that?" I demanded. Mark and I have an on-going battle about his tendency to overreact (which I'm fairly confident he's aware of—at least I hope so since this story will soon be part of public record). I was sure that whatever he had done had been a drastic overreaction and was about to cause some type of otherwise avoidable complication. It turns out I may have been wrong, but I wouldn't know that for a few more months. We squabbled back and forth for a minute before he hurried off the phone. The next time I heard from him was when they were in the hospital.

I answered the call to hear him crying. "What's going on?" I demanded. "Is Connor OK?"

"He's fine. I'm not. I can't go back in there," Mark told me.

"What do you mean you can't go back in there? You have to."

"I can't. You have to come here. I need your help," He explained.

"What are you talking about? You're coming home tomorrow. Why in the world would I fly there now just to fly back with you one day later?" Of course this line of reasoning made perfect sense to me, but was meaningless to Mark.

"I don't know what I'm doing. I don't know how to take care of him." And then with some more crying, "I think I almost killed him."

"You didn't almost kill him," I tried to reassure him, but I don't know that a glucagon shot was the best decision. Was he unconscious?"

"No, but he kept crashing," he explained. "No matter what I did, he just kept crashing. I didn't know what else to do."

And so would be our life for the following few months until Connor's completely uncontrollable numbers had us seriously concerned. There were times when he could eat up to eighty grams of carbs with little to no blood sugar spike—and the doctor was sure that he was well out of the honeymoon phase. We would go upwards of twelve hours without administering any insulin, because every time we gave it, his numbers would plummet again. While this may seem like a blessing on the surface, it is actually quite concerning because the body can quickly fall into DKA (even if blood glucose numbers are low) when there is an insufficient supply of insulin.

At this point, it was the start of a new school year, and I could barely focus on work because the majority of my time was spent on the phone with doctors—the endocrinologist multiple times per day: "I think his kidneys might be shutting down," he explained to me. "We need to run some tests." And the pediatrician: "Maybe he just keeps battling the flu—it's going around."

By this time we had transitioned Connor into a special education preschool class at the local elementary school. We were the second family in the state to be found eligible for nursing care during school hours, but it would only be provided if he attended a preschool program that was attached to one of the public elementary schools. And so special education it was. We were fortunate to be assigned a wonderfully caring nurse who treated him like her own son—Connor loved her! As things got more and more out of control with his numbers, we frequently found ourselves pulling him out of school. A number of times his nurse actually spent time with him at home (unpaid) so that she could assist my parents while I worked, and she even accompanied us to the doctor's office.

"He does not have the flu," she stressed to the pediatrician. "I've been working with him for over two months and I'm telling you that something else is going on."

We explained that the bouts of diarrhea and vomiting kept coming in waves, and even when Connor seemed otherwise well, digestive issues seemed to be an ongoing problem.

"Maybe we should check him for celiac," The doctor suggested.

I hated the thought of another diagnosis, but celiac sure seemed like a better alternative to kidney failure. "Let's do it," I said.

And so the pediatrician gave us a referral to a GI doctor to have him screened for celiac—a process which involves general anesthesia and a scope of the upper intestinal tract. In preparation for meeting with the new doctor, we had results of blood work sent over from the screening the endocrinologist had ordered for Connor over the summer (diabetics are generally given a preliminary blood screening each year for celiac and other autoimmune diseases because of their increased risk for developing such conditions).

It took less than 48 hours to hear back from the pediatrician. "I passed along your labs to the gastro and we talked about Connor's symptoms," he told me. "She said that while his numbers from the summer screening don't reflect an urgent medical condition, based on his digestive issues and your inability to stabilize his blood sugar, she's fairly confident that he has celiac." As I would learn only months later, his number was 39. In the grand scheme of things, 39 is not terribly high, but it is definitely a sign of trouble—as the members of my one support groups have taught me, anything over 20 is indicative of celiac, but numbers can skyrocket into the hundreds when the disease is left uncontrolled.

"Should we still plan to have him scoped?" I asked.

"No. She doesn't have an appointment available for him for a few months, and he would need to stay on gluten that entire time in order for the results to be accurate," he explained. "We both feel he should be taken off gluten immediately. If he does well on a gluten-free diet, you can feel confident in the diagnosis, but if you want absolute confirmation down the road, you can put him back on gluten in a few months and have him checked then."

"If the gluten free diet works for him, why would we put him back on gluten?" I asked.

"Because that's the only way to get a confirmed diagnosis," he told me. "For now, we both feel that it would be medically irresponsible to keep him on a gluten diet and put a medically unstable toddler under general anesthesia."

And just like that my world was rocked again—I had a medically unstable child who now not only had one chronic disease, but another that was sure to restructure everything I knew about feeding and caring for my son.

The initial diagnosis came in November of 2015. By January I had quit my full-time job at the high school and picked up some part-time lecturing hours at the college. There was just no way I could manage a regular full-time job and meet all of Connor's medical and dietary needs. After speaking with the doctor that day (our conversation had fortunately happened on a Friday afternoon), I did a lot of research on gluten-free living and joined my second favorite support group—Parents of Children with Celiac Disease and Type 1 Diabetes. Mark and I spent the entire weekend cleaning out the entire kitchen of everything that might contain gluten (right down to the bulk of our spices). The process was a slow one since we had to read every label and cross-check the majority of ingredients for possible association with gluten.

The changeover was tedious, but we were quickly rewarded for our efforts. We saw an almost immediate reduction in symptoms within the first week. His digestive issues cleared up, and his body started responding to carbohydrates in food again. We knew we had found our culprit.

Living with celiac is in some ways much more difficult than living with diabetes. With diabetes he can eat anything he wants, we just have to cover all of his food with a proper dose of insulin. With celiac disease, we have to worry about not only the food he eats, but everything he comes in contact with. This means that even dining out and giving him gluten-free food in a restaurant where non-GF food is served can pose a major health risk to him. And sometimes even nonfood items can cause problems. We learned that lesson the hard way when we landed ourselves back in the hospital one night because Connor was screaming of stomach pain. He was literally doubled over unable to keep his body in an upright position. We had let him play with play-dough earlier that day.

With both diseases we are constantly learning and re-configuring our management plan. We have good days, and downright terrible days. There are days when I just break down and cry because I am so completely physically and emotionally drained. But there are plenty of other days—when he's laughing and running around like a normal kid and all I can think of is how grateful I am that we caught his conditions in time to avoid any lasting effects and that we live in a time when disease management is much more advanced than it once was.

Update:

Roughly 5 years later we were told that the celiac diagnosis had possibly been a mistake. A new blood test revealed no indication of any type of disease. His numbers on the blood screening were actually zero--An indication of complete absence of disease. We opted to put Connor back on gluten for a couple of months so that we could go ahead with the "gold standard" of diagnostic tests to determine whether or not he truly had celiac. In those trial months Connor really lived it up! He thoroughly enjoyed being able to eat whatever his siblings ate. We saw some fluctuations in BG but attributed that to our new climate (we had recently moved from HI to CA). And he wasn't having the stomach cramping that he had experienced earlier, so we were really hopeful that the whole thing had been a big mistake. Until we learned that it wasn't. The endoscopy confirmed that he did in fact have celiac (and that the normal blood test results were reflective of our careful dietary management). It was determined that he had to immediately go back to a gluten-free lifestyle. Breaking that news to him was one of the hardest things for me to do because I knew that there would be no mystery for him in what the diagnosis meant. He has always considered celiac to be a much graver life-altering condition than diabetes.

Footnotes:

Normal ranges are somewhere around 100. DKA is short for Diabetic Ketoacidocis. According to the American Diabetes Association, "Diabetic ketoacidosis (DKA) is a serious condition that can lead to diabetic coma (passing out for a long time) or even death." When cells don't get the glucose they need for energy, the body begins to burn fat for energy, which produces ketones. - See more at: http://www.diabetes.org/living-with-diabetes/complications/ketoacidosis-dka.html#sthash.lUOZr3ZT.dpuf Pediatric Intensive Care Unit IBCLC stands for Internationally Board Certified Lactation Consultant One of the emergency devices parents are trained on in the hospital is a glucagon shot (similar in many ways to an EpiPen for individuals with severe allergies). The kit contains a large needle and an airtight vial of glucagon which keeps the product preserved until injected. While some parents administer "mini-shots" to help bring up low blood glucose in little kids who are unable to take in sufficient carbs on their own, most people reserve glucagon injections for severe emergencies when the diabetic individual has lost consciousness and can not be administered carbohydrates by mouth. The honeymoon phase is the period of time following diagnosis when a patient's body continues to make small, but irregular amounts of insulin. This period usually lasts about a year to eighteen months until the pancreas completely stops functioning altogether. For some people the honeymoon phase offers a more relaxed way to get used to managing diabetes as the diabetic patient can often go long stretches without any insulin supplementation at all. For others the time is found to be incredibly stressful because they are unsure when synthetic insulin will be needed and when it won't.

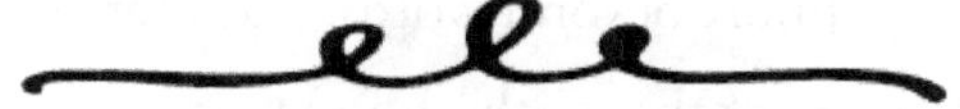

Nanny

When I asked my own mother to contribute to this project, I knew I was taking a risk. A risk that she would stir up old memories that I had successfully repressed, or would challenge certain truths that I had been holding onto that might not actually be as accurate as I wanted them to be. But I've come to terms with that possibility realizing that I am profoundly curious about how she sees my world, and more specifically how she views me as both a daughter and mother to her grandchildren. I also feel the need to honor her by sharing her story because the truth is I don't think I would have survived these past 2 ½ years without her support. Yes, my father, who has recently passed, served an active role in this process too. And yes, I have valued his love and support beyond words, but there's something about being the current bearer of the motherhood torch that made me need to know how I'm doing in the eyes of my own mom.

When I first started writing this book, I envisioned an entire chapter dedicated to the experiences of grandmothers, but I couldn't figure out a way to incorporate an entire chapter on "Voices from Grandmothers" without turning this work into a mini-encyclopedia. Maybe, at some point I will be able to give voice to the grandparent experience in a separate book. In the meantime, I am happy to be able to share my mother's story as an expansion on our collective experience caring for Connor.

As I surely mentioned in my own retelling of events from the past few years, my mother is a rock. I mean that metaphorically of course, but in some ways I feel it literally too. Maybe it's her Eastern European blood and sturdy frame. She's always hated her legs—more hardy than the long and lean ones that I inherited from my father's side of the family. And as she will attest, she has veins like ropes. She doesn't love this description of her, but for me, her daughter, it's part of what makes her so strong.

I'm quite the opposite of my mother. My build, my veins, everything. I have never given blood. Not because I don't want to, but because I really think that I'm more trouble than I'm worth for the nurses at the blood donation center. The times in my life that I've had to have blood drawn has always a huge hassle where they'd have to warm my arms with heated blankets and flood me full of liquids just to plump my veins up enough to get the sample they needed.

Not my mom. She gives blood all the time. She has even given platelets (because that's the kind of person she is), though I don't think she'll be repeating that experience anytime soon. They love her at the donation center because she actually has veins that look like ropes from which the blood flows freely, and she's more than happy to offer them up for the benefit of others. That's my mom—generous beyond words. Sturdy. Strong. Dependable.

This is why when I read her written words about my first phone call to her from the hospital (she graciously typed up her story for me on a day's notice), I started to cry: "I remember feeling faint, lightheaded, almost ready to pass out." We still didn't have an official diagnosis at that point, but the doctors were pretty confident that it was Type 1 diabetes. "Panic quickly set in," she explained.

On a subconscious level, I'm sure I always knew that my mother was capable of weakness, but it is something she rarely demonstrates, allowing me to believe that the center of her brain that controls such emotions was somehow muted at birth. But of course it wasn't. And every time that I call her crying, I'm sure she feels that tug of fear and ineptness that we all experience as mothers, but she puts it on the side so that she can be strong for me.

What I found most interesting in her story was her mention of missing her own mother's strength and knowledge at that moment when our call ended. "For many years I was spoiled by the fact that my mother was a doctor," she wrote. "Even though she lived in Europe and I was here in the United States, she was always my go-to person for anything related to medical questions. She was a font of knowledge, and always willing to lend an ear and give advice. How I missed her now!"

As mom explains, she went on to do the thing we all do in today's technology-driven world—she turned to Dr. Internet. "It was the only thing I could do," she says. "And so over the next several days, while Connor was hospitalized in Chicago's Children's Hospital, and I sat helpless 1,000 miles away in New York, I spent every free moment reading up on Diabetes." And as she learned, "Sometimes a little knowledge is a terrible thing! The more I read, the more scared I got, with so much varying and sometimes conflicting information out there!"

We've all been there. I know I certainly have—reading the online stories of how things can and most certainly will go terribly wrong. We all know it's crazy to make medical predictions for ourselves and loved ones based on things we read in chat rooms or on WebMd, but those sites just continue to draw us in and lock us there, as we desperately search for the golden nugget of information that will make everything come clear.

Unfortunately, the information she found online paled in comparison to some of the horrific things people said to her upon hearing the news of Connor's condition. After reading my version of her story, she called and said, "I just remembered something terrible that happened in those first early days. I guess it upset me so much that I just pushed it out of my mind." She was referring to a conversation she had had with an old acquaintance. The man was a retired physician—a very strong-minded one. I had met him several times while visiting with my parents, and he had always rubbed me the wrong way. Apparently, he hadn't worked on his people skills at all since my last encounter with him because when my mother ran into him and explained what was going on with Connor, he replied, "You know you have to prepare your daughter for the fact that he will die—probably within the year!" My mom remembers being so shocked by his statement that she walked away speechless, unable to find the words to reply.

Fortunately, we had all just seen each other a few weeks earlier, and she was able to draw on the positive images of him running and playing with his brothers and sisters. She calmly reassured herself that Connor couldn't really be that sick that he might actually die. "I remembered that Connor hadn't looked well over the visit," she remembers. "That he had looked pale and skinny compared to the rest of the grandkids. But I reassured myself that it was probably just the late fall cold weather, and all the kids coming home from school with all kinds of bugs." Her words mirror the thoughts that were going on in all of our heads at that point: Could he really have been sick for weeks without any of us picking up on it?

"I actually remember pulling up pictures from the Chicago visit on my computer while waiting for more news from Erin," she recalls. "Just to convince myself that I was wrong and that Connor had looked fine then. But there it was right in front of me. He looked pale and not really well. Now, in hindsight, everything started to come back to me. Erin telling me that Connor had lately started intentionally banging his head on the walls and floors, being cranky and wanting to nurse almost all the time...I now questioned how we could have missed all the signs. But how would we know what all these signs meant?"

And she's right. There had been so many signs leading up to his actual diagnosis. I remember casually mentioning to the pediatrician (during my older daughter's well visit) that Connor had started pounding his head on hard surfaces whenever he was angry. She told me that he was probably doing it out of frustration—being the youngest in a family of four kids is no joke for a little one. She told me that I should put him in a safe place (like a padded crib or playpen) when he got like that so that he could get the tantrum over with without seriously injuring himself. If only we had known then that his little body was screaming out in pain from the inside.

As my mom reflects on our earliest conversations surrounding his diagnosis, she remembers the jolt of realization: "After those first early conversations, while I was desperately waiting for more news, everything from the recent past came into sharp focus."

"And just like when I first heard mention of the word diabetes", my mom shares, "My mind flashed to my niece. Some thirty-eight years earlier, she had been diagnosed with what was then called Juvenile Diabetes. She was twelve years old at the time, and the diabetes supposedly came as the result of a virus. At that time, none of us realized how very serious this diagnosis was. I was quite young then, in my early-twenties, and I still remember thinking, 'What a pain in the neck. Now she will have to take insulin shots twice a day forever!' How little did I know then—it should only be that simple!"

And my mom would soon see what a pain in the neck caring for a Type 1 toddler could be. She spent the month of January with us (the month following his diagnosis) so she could help us settle into our new home on Maui and so my husband Mark and I could get our acts together with the new routine—I was now the working parent, back to full-time teaching, and he was taking over the responsibilities of stay-at-home parenting until we could find suitable childcare.

"After Erin and Mark decided to go through with their plans to move back to Maui," my mom remembers, "my husband spent hours trying to secure an apartment for the family." Most Maui agents are hesitant to rent to people off island and mandate that at least one family member be present to inspect the property and sign the papers beforehand. This usually means that people moving from off-island have to plan to stay in a hotel for a few weeks while they look for a place to live. We all knew that this type of arrangement wouldn't be possible, now that we had the added stress of trying to manage Connor's new medical needs.

Unfortunately, with me and Mark hospital-bound, trying to make sense of our new roles and responsibilities as parents of a diabetic toddler, we were in no position to spend hours on the phone arguing with rental agents. This is where my dad stepped in. Eventually he struck up a conversation with one of the agents, letting the man know that they might be interested in buying property by year's end and that if all went well with the rental, the guy might see a nice commission from the deal. That was all it took—we officially had a home to move into.

"Unfortunately," as my mom remembers, "the rental agent forgot all about us, and when we finally showed up on island, it took several hours to find his boss to come unlock the apartment. The kids and I had spent the past several hours dealing with the stomach flu, and we had the added worry of needing to get Connor's insulin into refrigeration."

This really was a nightmare. My mom and all of the kids (including Connor) has spent the entire trip throwing up on the plane, in the airport lounges between flights, and in the hotel room that we stayed in on the first night—we had arrived on island on New Year's Eve and couldn't move into our new place until New Year's Day.

"I still remember my head over the toilet while listening to the fireworks go off," my mom recalls. It was definitely a holiday like none other. "We were sick, tired, and scared," she points out. "By the next day, Connor's insulin had been without real refrigeration for over twenty-four hours and we didn't know what to do. It was baking in our luggage, and we were panicking." Eventually, we did manage to get in touch with the owner of the rental agency who was able to grant us access to the apartment, but in all the chaos of the preceding weeks, we had overlooked our responsibility of calling to have electric turned on for our arrival, and now we were stuck with none.

"Our phones were dead, and we had no way to charge them," my mom explains. "There was no furniture to sit on, and we had no way to keep anything cool. We had bought air mattresses at K-Mart that morning so that we'd have something comfortable to sleep on, but we couldn't even inflate them because we had no electricity."

We were starting to question the practicality of our situation when the upstairs neighbors got home and came to our rescue. "They strung an extension cord out the window for us, lent us a lamp, and got us some ice, and that's how we survived the night. A few days later Mark arrived and so did our container with all of the furniture—things seemed to be improving."

My mom only stayed a few weeks at that point. My dad had stayed behind in our Chicago place, getting things straightened up so it could be put on the market and then spent two days driving alone through an ice storm back to New York. My mom met him there where they reviewed the options.

"Seeing how difficult the situation was for Erin and Mark, we made the decision to put our house in New York up for sale, and relocate full-time to Maui. This was not an easy decision, considering how involved we were in our local art community and how settled we were. For a while we played with the idea of living half the year in New York and half the year in Hawaii. Looking back at that now, I realize just how impossible that would have been, and how unworkable."

In March, my parents flew back to spend some time with us and discuss long-range plans. We were only on a six-month lease, and with six people squeezed into a tiny two-bedroom apartment, we weren't eager to renew. My parents decided to buy a house (Mark and I were in no financial position to buy one for ourselves) so that we could mutually pay into a family investment rather than lining the pockets of some far-away landlord or rental agency. I love that my parents think in such practical terms and that they were able to turn that sense into something that made life manageable for me, Mark, and the kids.

We moved into our new house in June of that same year, and Mark spent several weeks of the summer renovating the cottage on the property so that it could be rented out and used as supplemental income for my parents. Two months later, my parents joined us on island and started looking for a condo for themselves. In just a short period of time, things seemed to be falling into place nicely. As I review this story (years after initially writing it), I am reminded of how important it is to solve the problems of the moment, rather than trying to solve the unknown problems of the future.

"When we first arrived in August," my mom remembers, "I still had the erroneous idea that Connor's diabetes was a disease that could be managed by several well-timed injections each day. The reality of just how difficult it is to manage, especially with a still mostly nonverbal 2-year-old, quickly set in. I read everything I could get my hands on, but nothing prepared me for the actual experience of taking this child under my care, even for a limited amount of time."

By the time my parents officially moved to Maui, we had established Connor with one of the local nursery schools so that Mark and I could both work full time—a necessity in this beautiful, but expensive, slice of paradise. The women at the center were wonderful and worked hard to take good care of him, but there were frequent issues with out-of-range blood sugars and insulin pump failures, and my parents quickly became the emergency contacts for when Mark and I were at work.

"One day shortly after we arrived," my mom remembers with some frustration, "I offered to take Connor to the pediatrician, so Erin would not have to take a day off (there had been too many of those already). The Medical Center we used then was more than 12 miles away, so the trip took some time on the slow Maui roads. After waiting almost 45 minutes for the doctor to show up, Connor started falling apart. It was clear he was not feeling well, and I needed to measure his blood sugar. I thought I knew how to use the meter and lancing device, but no matter how hard I tried, I could not make it work. I was in a total panic, and asked for some help from the nursing staff. It turns out none of the nurses were familiar with the device, and one finally offered to see if they had any meters and lancets that they might know how to use."

"By this time, Connor was screaming, I was crying, and the doctor finally sailed in, offering this bit of wisdom, without having any numbers to go by: 'We have some crackers here, just give him some, he is probably just hungry!' The nurse finally got his blood sugar checked, and he was almost 400! Giving him crackers would have been a disaster. Needless to say, that was the last time we visited that doctor."

I still remember that day. I was in my classroom when I got the call—this time the tables were turned and it was me that sat helpless on the other end of the line, wishing there was something I could do to help my mom, but knowing that I couldn't offer anything other than those same well-intentioned but useless words, "Don't worry. Everything will be fine."

In another instance, my mom recalls feeling totally overwhelmed and unable to act under the pressure: "The next time I had Connor with me for a couple of hours to do our weekly shopping at Costco. By this time, I had practiced pricking his finger and checking his numbers, so I felt a bit more confident. I checked his blood sugar, and the meter read 220. All of a sudden, everything I knew just completely evaporated from my brain. What does it mean: 220? Is that high? Is that low? Do I give him an insulin shot, or do I give him something to eat? I remember being so totally at a loss, despite all of my mental preparation. I called Erin in panic, and it was as if we had reversed our roles again. She was the mother and I was the child. She calmly talked me through the next steps, and reassured me."

These two events happened when we were still in our first year after Connor's diagnosis, so there were plenty of moments when we all felt at a loss for what to do. As time has passed, we've all gained more confidence in our ability to manage crisis situations.

"Some days are better than others," my mom says. "I remember the very first time that I felt somewhat reassured that with proper care, Connor would be able to live a good life. We were having repair work done on our garden sprinkler system, and the repairman, in his early forties, good-looking and fit, noticed Connor's pump. He pulled his shirt up, showing us that he uses the same one. He said he was diagnosed at twelve years of age, and told us just how tough it was going through the first years, as a teenager with diabetes, and how good his life is now. He laughed that his wife does more worrying than he does. A few days later, at the kids' swim meet, a similar thing happened. The father of one of the swimmers, noticing Connor's pump, came to us to tell us he has had Type 1 Diabetes for many years, and to reassure us that life can be pretty good even with the condition. 'It is just so important to take good care of yourself,' he told us. 'And even then, there will be good days and bad days.'"

"This conversation led me to look up names of athletes who live with Type 1 diabetes," my mom recalls. "As it turns out, there were so many names—so many big name athletes! Jay Cutler, for one... quarterback for

Mark's favorite NFL team, the Chicago Bears. Every day, I tell myself that Connor can and will grow up to be someone special!"

We all believe that's true—it's what we have to believe to get through the day-to-day life of managing a disease that requires giving multiple daily injections and restricting or forcing food on a toddler who can barely even pronounce the word Diabetes.

I'd like to say that the days have gotten easier—I guess in many ways they have. But they are not easy. There are so many nights where I put my head down on the pillow and think, thank goodness that day is behind me. But there are wonderful days too, and having my parents here to share those days is priceless. I know that if they were still living in New York, they would still function as my rock, but there would be no way for me to share the beautiful sunsets and carefree afternoons at the pool with them and the kids, and it's those moments—those flashes of normalcy—that make everything ok.

Chapter Three

Breastfeeding at Diagnosis

The stories in this chapter represent the diversity of experiences of women who were still nursing their infants or toddlers at the time of diagnosis. Until recently, the percentage of babies diagnosed with Type 1 Diabetes at a time when they were still receiving milk from their mothers was quite small. This is partially because extended breastfeeding rates in this country are relatively low compared to other parts of the world, and because until recently, children were often well beyond infancy by the time they were diagnosed.

Breastfeeding rates are now on the rise (a wonderful thing!), and unfortunately so are the rates of Type 1 diagnoses in younger and younger children. The incidence of Type 1 diabetes is increasing roughly 3% each year, with a current rough estimate of 15,000 children diagnosed annually, and children seem to be getting diagnosed younger and younger. This shared increase in trends has led to a larger number of women and babies finding themselves in the predicament of trying to figure out how to incorporate breastfeeding into a diabetes management plan.

Because hospital policies vary and individual doctors and nurses have differing levels of understanding when it comes to the benefits of breastfeeding, the support breastfeeding mothers will receive from the endocrinology team in their hospital is primarily based on luck. Some women are urged to immediately wean with the idea that a diet void of breastmilk will make the process of counting carbohydrates cleaner and neater—this misconception will be addressed in several places throughout the stories that follow.

Fortunately, some women find themselves in the care of wonderfully supportive medical teams, with doctors and nurses experienced in the fine art of incorporating breastfeeding into the diabetes management program. The experiences of these women can serve as reassurance for those who are struggling to find support, that yes, it can be done!

A Note Before You Jump In:

Theresa and Daphne's Story (the first one in this chapter) is interrupted by a number of author commentary sections. I apologize to anyone who is bothered by the interruption in storytelling. I used this introductory story as a space to share some background information that I thought might prove useful to understanding all of the mothers' stories throughout this book. If you find such interruptions annoying, you might consider jumping ahead and reading those boxed-off sections (titled ~ A Note From Erin ~) before you jump into the narratives.

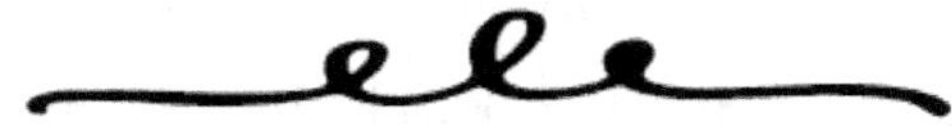

Theresa & Daphne: Fighting Back Against Demands to Wean

Like most of the other women in this book, I first got to know Theresa through an online support group. Theresa had been at this game a bit longer than I had—her daughter Daphne was diagnosed roughly nine months before my son Connor, in March of 2012. That means that by the time I approached Theresa about this project, it had already been over four years since those early days spent in the hospital with a little baby. Fortunately, like me, Theresa had felt the need to process her emotions through writing and speaking out. She had written an article for the Breastfeeding Center of San Diego, created a beautiful YouTube video highlighting some of the challenges and triumphs of the first year, and conducted an interview with the hospital where Daphne was diagnosed long before I ever reached out to her. Of course, I was overjoyed to find such a treasure-trove of details to help me in writing up her story, but more importantly, I was inspired by her determination to record such a significant time in her daughter's life.

While the experiences that Theresa has recorded might be flavored more bitter than sweet, the overall message that Daphne will receive as she grows into a young woman is that she is strong and capable of anything. I hope that in sharing the story of these two courageous females, I will inspire others to find strength in writing, video-taping, photographing—whatever it takes to capture these precious moments before they're lost to the mix of clouded memories.

"It started with a cold around Christmas time," Theresa explained as she started me on her journey through the past—such a simple little thing that so many families with young children suffer through around the holidays.

Only this time young Daphne didn't seem to be getting any better. "She was asking for water a lot," but as Theresa recalls with an ironic sense of comedy that only time allows, "Since Daphne had just learned to say 'water', we thought she was just excited about her new word." Over the course of a few short weeks, Daphne had lost a lot of weight (which isn't good when you're only nineteen months old) and it seemed to be getting harder and harder for her to breathe. That's when Theresa and her husband, Luke, decided it was time to see the doctor.

They took Daphne to her regular pediatrician, Theresa's worry intensifying as Daphne struggled for each breath. The nurse came into the room and immediately hooked her up to a nebulizer. It didn't seem to be working.

The doctor walked in and started asking questions. "When did the symptoms begin?"... "Have you noticed anything else out of the usual?"

Theresa recounted as many details as she could recall. "I've noticed that her skin has felt a little funny lately," she mentioned. The doctor asked for a glucometer to be brought in immediately. "Within seconds, a pin prick revealed a small drop of blood on Daphne's slender finger, followed by a countdown and then a number on the screen: 580—a blood glucose level ore than five times normal.

"Your daughter had Type 1 Diabetes," the doctor explained. "She's breathing that way because she is in diabetic shock." After excusing herself for a moment, the doctor returned to alert Theresa to the plan.

"I've called Children's Hospital and the doctors are expecting you in the ER. I would call an ambulance but iw will be faster if you drive. You need to leave right now."

"How did this happen?" Theresa asked. "Was it something we did?"

~ A Note From Erin ~

I remember asking this same question myself. And Theresa and I are not alone. Parents are often quick to blame themselves when their child gets hurt or sick, but the sense of guilt is even more pronounced when faced with a chronic medical condition such as diabetes. Because of the growing Type 2 epidemic in this country—often a reflection of poor diet and exercise practices—doctors are quick to remind parents that a healthy diet, in combination with activities that keep kids off the couch and away from video games is essential in helping prevent diabetes. This catchall phrase leads most people to believe that diabetes is a singular disease, and that Type 1 can somehow be prevented—or caused.

I suppose in some way the two are similar in that according to the American Diabetes Association, diabetes is "a problem with your body that causes blood glucose (sugar) to rise higher than normal." But the link ends there. The difference in diseases—both causes and effects—is vast. Unfortunately, parents are still left thinking that they did something to cause their child's condition, and as the years go by, the person living with the disease often starts to hide it from others for fear of being judged as irresponsible.

~ Continued Note ~

Type 2—the type of diabetes that affects nearly ninety percent of all diabetics, and thus gets the most attention—is what is referred to by doctors as "insulin-resistant" diabetes. In other words, the body generally produces plenty of insulin (a hormone) on its own, but because the body has been mistreated for so long, it can no longer make use of it to effectively process carbohydrates in the body. For many years, the condition was most commonly diagnosed in adults 35 and over (thus the distinction of "Juvenile Diabetes" for Type 1). But with the rising incidence of obesity in American children, Type 2 is presenting younger and younger, making the term juvenile applicable to both.

Type 1, on the other hand, affects about 10-15 percent of diabetics and usually presents itself in childhood. Fortunately, the classification of "juvenile" is starting to fade away with the rise of pediatric Type 2 cases and an increasing number of grownups now being diagnosed with Type 1. I say this is fortunate because in the past, too many adults were misdiagnosed as Type 2 due to assumptions made based on age. As I mentioned before, the two diseases are quite different, and proper diagnosis is essential in effectively managing the disease.

**I know this has been a long enough sidebar from Theresa's story, but if you can stick with me a few more minutes, I promise there's a point to all of this! But if you'd like to get back to her story, she picks up again on page 61.

~ Final Portion Of This Note (I Promise!) ~

Unlike Type 2, Type 1 is the result of an autoimmune disease (usually), caused when the body sees the pancreas as a foreign body and attacks it. I say this is usually the case because there have been instances where the pancreas has been destroyed by physical forces such as an accident, and the result is the same: Once the pancreas has been destroyed, it can no longer produce the essential hormone that allows the body to effectively process carbohydrates. Type 1 diabetics are thus referred to as "Insulin Dependent" because they require daily injections of insulin in order to turn food into energy.

There are over 80 types of autoimmune diseases, including Lupus, Rheumatoid Arthritis, Hashimoto, and Addison's. The exact reasons why one individual develops an autoimmune disease and another doesn't is still somewhat of a mystery to the medical community, though current research supports a theory that these diseases are triggered by a combination of factors (such as genetics, environmental irritants, and bacterial or viral infections) rather than just one thing. What is clear is that parents can do everything right, and their child can still get the disease—it is certainly nobody's fault.

~ End of Note—Phew! ~

And of course, Theresa's doctor told her as much. Just as other doctors have told their patients countless times, but in that moment, emotions seem to weigh heavier than reason.

"With those words"—the diabetes diagnosis—Theresa explains, "My life changed forever. "When you take your child—your baby barely over a year and a half old—to the doctor for heavy breathing, the last thing you expect to hear is that they have an incurable disease and are fighting for their life."

But that's exactly what they were doing. This was a race against time to save Daphne's life, and they were just at the starting line. And so off they sped.

It was a nice hospital—one of the top in San Diego. Even in March, there was a vibrant green lawn and palm trees at the front door. They were greeted by a tall clock tower at the front and a big building built completely of glass to the side—like a castle for a princess. Only this castle was in the business of taking care of severely sick children, and Daphne was about to become one of its newest special guests. By the time they arrived, she was lapsing in and out of consciousness and her condition was quickly deteriorating.

"Luke [Theresa's husband] drove 80mph down the freeway and made it there in 15 minutes," Theresa remembers. When we got to the ER entrance, he threw the car keys at the attendant and ran past all of the other people in the waiting room. I remember all the nasty looks from all the people waiting as we ran by."

Luke laid his little girl on the waiting gurney, and the emergency crew immediately set to work. They quickly stripped Daphne of her street clothes and changed her into a hospital gown. It was cute, with orange tigers, but designed mostly for function—to accommodate the vast array of wires and tubes that would soon be attached to her body. She was transferred to the emergency care center where doctors began working feverishly to stabilize her condition.

They inserted a catheter for urine and struggled to start an IV to administer fluids. It took multiple attempts to finally get the IV going and at one point, the nurse pushed a chair under Theresa who nearly fainted from the shock. "I eventually had to leave the room so Daphne wouldn't see me panic," Theresa explains.

~ A Note From Erin ~

Unfortunately, this is the state in which many infant and toddler diabetics enter the hospital, leaving parents to watch as helpless bystanders, while doctors and nurses scurry to save a young life. When diabetes is left untreated (as is often the case with young children who can't express their discomfort in the early stages of the disease), it eventually leads to DKA, which is a life-threatening condition.

In this condition, the body struggles to sustain itself, breaking down body fat to convert it to energy (which is why Daphne had gotten so skinny). In the process, chemicals called ketones are produced and build up in the blood. As a result of the body's effort to rid itself of the ketones, the person in DKA finds themself perpetually thirsty while experiencing the constant urge to urinate. This frequent urination (a telltale sign of diabetes) helps the body to flush ketones, but also leads to a life-threatening state of dehydration.

When young children first arrive at the hospital in this state, the emergency team's first order of business—before they can even begin to think about managing blood glucose levels—is to get the child rehydrated. Unfortunately, young children can dehydrate so quickly that their veins begin to collapse. Veins in the arms and hands, which serve as common sites for IV hook-up, wind up inaccessible and more drastic measures, such as delivery through the jugular in the neck, or veins in the scalp, have to be attempted. The experience of watching doctors try to treat a young child in DKA is often quite traumatizing.

~ End Note ~

Unfortunately, Daphne was in such an extremely critical state, that the medical team asked if the family would like to have a visit from the chaplain. Theresa was forced to confront the fact that her daughter might not make it through the night.

"I feel like I've forgotten so much between the time we entered the hospital and the moment the nurse shoved that chair under me," Theresa says, "but I do remember the IV. After they finally got it in, it just started bleeding and wouldn't stop—it bled all night. It was the night before St. Patrick's Day and her arm was wrapped in a green splint with shamrocks on it. The blood just soaked through the whole thing so it was a mess of green and dried brown blood."

Fortunately, the family was able to move out of the emergency ward and into the ICU Step-Down department, where they shared a double room with another family. "Once they had Daphne stabilized," Theresa recalls, "she just cried all night. I felt terrible and kept apologizing to the other family."

It was a small room with little space for moving or comfortably resting. Theresa spent most of that first night with her body partially tucked inside Daphne's hospital crib. The combination of stress and lack of sleep started to wear on Theresa. "I just remember staring out the window at the rain all night," she shares. "At some point it became morning, but I couldn't even tell because it was so dreary"—an eerie reflection of her mood.

Because of Daphne's delicate state, she was not allowed to eat or nurse. "My daughter was barely conscious, was in pain and terrified while she was awake, and I could not even hold her because she wanted to nurse," Theresa explains. "I hope no other mama has to experience the excruciating helplessness you feel in a situation like that. Our children's hospital has no lactation consultants and by the time they could find a pump for me, we had already skipped about 7 or 8 feedings. I was scared to death and in physical pain myself."

Regardless of the reason, Daphne needed the comfort of breastfeeding that she had come to rely on, and Theresa desperately needed relief for her worsening engorgement. Theresa's friend, an IBCLC, had tried, over the phone, to explain how to do hand-compressions to express some milk, but Theresa couldn't make it work. Her sense of urgency was intensifying.

While overall breastfeeding rates and duration of breastfeeding are much higher in other countries, such frequent nursing by a child this age is uncommon in the US. Even for mothers who choose to allow their child to "nurse on demand" and practice "child-led weaning", most experience a decrease in nursing sessions by the time the child hits a year old and becomes more interested in solid foods. Like Daphne, my son was still nursing frequently at 15 months and barely taking in any solids. I've often wondered if these little ones chose breastmilk over solids as a defense mechanism, knowing that their bodies couldn't handle the variety of carbohydrates in common table food.

While Daphne's physical status seemed to be slowly but steadily improving, the emotional state of both mother and daughter was at great risk. Without lactation consultants to advocate on her behalf, Theresa was left to fight for herself, and without research or professionals to support her claims, she had a nearly impossible time of convincing the medical team that she should not only be allowed to nurse her daughter but that in fact, it was what she needed to do more than anything.

"When we were finally given the okay for her to eat, I had to fight tooth and nail to be able to breastfeed her," Theresa explains. "The doctors finally consented to her having breast milk, but because she was not a tiny baby, the doctors did not think it was important. They told me that [I had to pump and that] she absolutely had to drink from a cup or bottle."

Unfortunately, many medical professionals are unaware of the benefits of breastfeeding beyond a year and consider the practice something that is easily dispensed of. What they don't realize is that in addition to the significant benefits of breastfeeding a child into toddlerhood (both nutritionally and emotionally), there are equally significant risks to abrupt weaning—especially during times of extreme stress.

Fortunately, Theresa was well aware of the impact that her choice—to continue breastfeeding or abruptly wean—would have on them both. "No mother should ever have to beg to be able to feed her baby. It took hearing our daughter scream and sob hysterically for the doctor to finally take pity on us and let me breastfeed her. As I held my tiny girl in my arms, it was the first time I began to feel like there was a possibility that she would be okay."

As the days went on, people sent cards and stuffed animals to make Daphne feel better. She even had her best friend, a nice big giraffe named Sophie, to keep her company in her hospital crib. As Theresa says, "you do not expect the comfort a hand-sewn pillowcase made by a hospital volunteer can bring," but it does. The little presents and simple acts of compassion make those early days of hospital care just bearable enough to endure, but still harsh enough to remind you that the critical care ward is not a place you want to hang out in for long.

Daphne's crib had metal bars all around. There were wires, tubes, and beeping electronics everywhere, and now their most basic daily practice was being threatened. Even after Theresa was allowed to nurse Daphne that one time, she was urged to begin the weaning process. Everyone wanted to go home—especially Theresa.

Eventually, Daphne's condition improved enough that by week's end, they were prepped for hospital release. Once doctors had her blood sugar stabilized and a good idea of how much insulin Daphne would require, she didn't need to be on the hospital's machines anymore. But taking care of a child with diabetes is very hard work and there is a lot for parents to learn before they can take over the responsibility for themselves.

~ A Note From Erin ~

According to an article published in the National Library of Medicine's Pediatric Child Health, Children are often well enough for discharge within 2-4 days of initial diagnosis, but there is concern for the ongoing training of parents—especially in regard to hypoglycemic prevention and treatment. As the authors explain, young children are often started on extremely low doses of insulin to help minimize the risk of hypoglycemia, and the amount is slowly increased over time. In other words, the formula is not "perfected" when the family leaves the hospital, and the ratios will consistently be adjusted as the child grows.

What I appreciated most about this article was their mention of insulin management, specifically in regard to babies who are still breastfeeding. At no time in the article did the authors—a team of doctors and nurses—suggest that weaning was necessary or even advisable. They simply indicated that insulin ratios would need to be adjusted as dietary patterns evolve.

~ Continued Note ~

A notable difference in the management plan for young infants and toddlers, compared to older children, is that insulin is often administered post-meal so that calculations can be made based on what was actually eaten, rather than what was expected to be eaten. As children age, and intake can be better predicted, parents are usually advised to administer insulin before eating (known as "pre-bolusing") so that the insulin has a chance to release in the body. This is because the sugars from most carbohydrate-rich foods enter the bloodstream at a much faster rate than artificial insulin.

As time goes on, parents become increasingly comfortable knowing which foods will cause blood sugar spikes in their little ones and are likely to be eaten completely (such as birthday cake) and start incorporating pre-bolusing strategies into the care plan. The most important thing to remember is that the whole process is based on continuous learning and fine-tuning. To expect perfect, steady numbers in the early weeks and months following discharge just sets the parents up for feelings of failure.

In our case, the one thing our endocrinologist told us as we prepared to leave the hospital that last day was to "remember that there is no mistake you can't fix." He then went on to share a story about a young child who broke into his insulin pump and administered a full week's worth of insulin to himself within a matter of seconds. The parents called the doctor hysterical, afraid the child would go into hypoglycemic shock.

~ Continued Note ~

He went on to explain, "I told the parents to keep giving him steady amounts of simple sugars to balance out the insulin and to watch him carefully for the next 24 hours. Then I told them to put a padlock on the pump bag so it wouldn't happen again."

We were lucky to have such a calm and compassionate doctor. Through that one story he let us know that no matter how badly we thought we'd screwed up (which was certain to happen at some point), we could always call for advice and never be made to feel stupid for our mistakes. To this day I tell other new parents that the best resource in their diabetes toolbox is quick access to a caring doctor who treats them with respect.

~ End Erin's Note ~

As the final hospital days came to a close for the family, Theresa and her husband Luke studied diligently, learning how to care for Daphne on their own. They practiced giving shots on a practice pad (this, or on a little squishy orange, is the way most parents learn how to manage a syringe before they start practicing on their own child) and learned how to calculate doses. They learned about things like "covering carbs" and "correction doses" for times when Daphne's blood sugar gets too high, and they practiced mixing glucagon shots for times when Daphne's blood sugar might be too low and she is unconscious or otherwise incapable of ingesting carbohydrates by mouth. They practiced taking the needle cap off and putting it back on carefully so that they wouldn't accidentally prick their own fingers and learned the proper order for mixing insulin in a syringe and which one to give when. Daphne even practiced checking her giraffe's blood sugar. But most importantly, Theresa learned how to estimate carbohydrate intake during nursing sessions so that breastfeeding could remain a regular part of their daily routine.

"Eventually, we were able to meet with the hospital's diabetes dietician who helped me calculate the average amount of milk I produced per feeding," Theresa recalls. "We looked at the amount of milk I was able to express with a pump and then by using the general amount of carbohydrates contained in breastmilk, we were able to determine a rough estimate for carbohydrates per feeding. Together we came up with a plan to space out her feedings as much as possible to keep her blood glucose stable. The dietician was a lifesaver and a champion for us! She spoke to our doctor on our behalf and convinced him that including breastfeeding as part of our daughter's nutrition was in her best interest. The doctor has since become supportive."

~ A Note From Erin ~

Managing diabetes on a day-to-day basis is a lot of work, and most parents leave the hospital scared about their ability to do a good job in their new roles as medical caretakers. They wonder if they'll be able to remember all the steps in each process or if they'll sleep through the 3am alarm when it's time to get up and check blood sugar again. They balk at the idea of pricking their baby's fingers ten times (or more) in a 24 hour period, and they cry over the thought of pinning their little one down three, four, and five times each day to give the life-saving shot they know they need to give. Parents enter the hospital feeling confident in their ability to love, nurture, and comfort their child, but leave feeling overwhelmed by the fact that love now sometimes looks more like torture.

~ Continued Note ~

The fact that so many nursing mothers are unnecessarily stripped of the one tool that they have at their disposal to comfort their child in times of stress is unfortunate. What seems like a simple change in routine, "You have to wean them eventually anyway, right?" is actually a terrible blow at an already overwhelming time of upheaval. Many moms who are encouraged (or at least allowed) to continue nursing find that nursing provides a wonderful source of comfort and distraction during times of injections, finger sticks, and medical equipment site changes.

Some also find that nighttime nursing sessions can help ward off the middle-of-the-night lows that little ones often suffer. In the case of severe lows, a faster-acting source of carbs (such as juice) is sometimes needed, but with the carb count of an average nursing session calculated to be roughly 10-15 grams, it often substitutes nicely for "between meal snacks" that are otherwise prescribed by doctors.

~ End Erin's Note ~

As Theresa explains, "Continuing breastfeeding brought my daughter so much comfort in the months of learning to live with multiple injections and painful finger-prick blood tests. It was something normal and peaceful for both of us during a stressful time of adjustment. It supported her overall health. It was a perfect source of nutrition for her combined with solids and was amazing for bringing her blood glucose back up to a safe level if she began to drop low at night."

As days turned to weeks and months, Theresa quickly took on added roles such as that of bookkeeper, keeping stringent records that could rival any accountant. She kept precise records of carb intake, insulin distribution, and blood glucose levels among other things. The stress of such added burdens can become overwhelming for many moms who already feel taxed by the regular responsibilities of managing the household and possibly even work outside the home. Theresa strongly believes that her ability to continue nursing for the year beyond initial diagnosis helped her keep stress levels in check and maintain a sense of normalcy that otherwise is often lost to this demanding disease.

There are actually more than 2 types, but that is a complicated discussion outside the scope of this book.

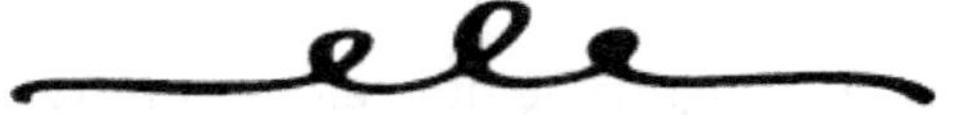

Brittany and Norah: Overcoming Obstacles and Push-back

Like Theresa, I met Brittany online, but this time it was the mom who reached out to me, instead of the other way around. I got a private message from her one day saying that she had come across my post about writing a book sharing the experiences of babies nursing past diagnosis. "Until I found this page [Diapers and Diabetes]," she told me, "I couldn't find anything online about breastfeeding a diabetic child." While I've had some non-breastfeeding moms jump at the chance to join this project, it seems that the women who were faced with the possibility of having to abruptly wean their infant during a time of such heightened stress are the ones that are most desperate to share their stories.

This is not a statement against formula-feeding mothers, or mothers who had already long passed the weaning stage—it is simply an acknowledgment that breastfeeding is a precious and intimate process, and when women choose to breastfeed, they generally envision a gradual transition from exclusive feeding in the infancy stage, to a system of partial nursing supplemented by other food sources in later months (or even years), and eventually tapering off when the timing seems right for both mom and baby. Any change in that plan—most commonly brought on by abrupt weaning—can be highly traumatic for the mother and her nursling. This is not unique to the world of diabetes. Sometimes even just the possibility of such a radical shift or a temporary break in nursing (as in instances when the mother has to undergo a procedure) can be highly stressful for a woman. I believe Brittany's urge to share her story comes from both the need to process such powerful emotions, as well as a compulsion to prevent other women from having to deal with such an unnecessary added burden at an already difficult time.

Baby Norah's story begins like many others—a stomach bug that just didn't want to go away. At nine-months old, she was past the delicate infant stage, and with two-plus years of motherhood under her belt (thanks to big brother Aaron who was at the time nearing two and a half), Brittany felt comfortable relying on nature's medicine (breastmilk) to get her baby through the weekend until they could visit the doctor on Monday morning. After all, there was no fever, and while more irritable than usual, Norah was alert and able to nurse frequently throughout the day and night. She was wetting her diapers, which offered her parents some sense of reassurance—"At least she isn't dehydrated" they reassured themselves. At least that's what they believed.

Unfortunately, many parents make the common mistake of equating wet diapers with proper hydration. What they don't realize is that when the body voids fluids from both ends of the body (as with a child who is both urinating and vomiting) it is actually a sign of distress. As my pediatrician explained to me just after Connor's diagnosis, children who have the flu will vomit, but will have minimum urine output because all fluids are lost orally. When a child loses fluids both through urination and vomiting, they quickly become severely dehydrated. This is what leads to the sunken eyes that so many parents describe as their first noticeable warning sign of trouble.

As the diapers mounted and Norah's condition worsened, Brittany and her husband Nathan struggled to comfort an increasingly distressed baby girl, while desperately trying to keep up with an energetic two-year-old and managing the responsibilities of the house.

"You go to work," Brittany told an exhausted Nathan on Monday morning. "I'll let you know how things go with the doctor." And with a quick kiss, he was out the door. Neither of them could possibly have imagined the whirlwind that would follow in the hours ahead.

Brittany hung up the phone with the doctor's receptionist, and although it broke her heart to put her little girl down, she rationalized that Norah would be ok while she took a minute to get dressed before the visit—after all, Norah's crib was only steps from the dresser. In the few minutes that she took to tend to her own needs—for what seemed like the first time in days—Norah's condition quickly deteriorated. Brittany recalls walking back to the crib to console her fussy baby, and in an instant knowing in her heart that something was horribly wrong. "Her normally rosy, pink cheeks were sunken deep and her usually bright eyes were dark and unresponsive. Her breaths were deep and labored, exposing her delicate skeletal frame beneath her little sleeper."

As Brittany watched the little blue cherries on Norah's jammies rise and fall with each labored breath, she knew that neither one of them could manage a car ride to the doctor. It was becoming increasingly obvious that Norah needed immediate care and Brittany was in no condition to drive.

"Nathan, you have to come home," she urged her husband over the phone. "Norah is getting worse. I'm calling for an ambulance. You have to come home now."

As Brittany explained to Jeff Kelly in an interview for the Akron Children's Hospital 2015 Radio-thon, "At that point we thought it was something respiratory." Gripped by fear that if she took her eyes off Norah, the sick infant would drift into a sleep from which she would never awaken, Brittany called 911 and counted the minutes until the ambulance's arrival—eight to be exact.

In those excruciating minutes that it took the ambulance to arrive, Norah's body grew limp in her mother's arms. She was slipping into a diabetic coma and it was all Brittany could do to keep her awake. "Please Norah. Please stay awake."

The paramedics immediately administered oxygen and did a quick assessment as they readied young Nora for her transport to the hospital. "Her heart rate and pulse are stable for now" they assured, "but you have to keep her awake."

With a combined sense of relief and absolute terror, Brittany climbed up into the ambulance and took Norah's side.

"Norah sweetheart—Stay awake for mommy. Please baby—just keep looking at mommy."

As the ambulance raced off—eerily quiet without its sirens blaring—Brittany continued to lovingly coax her baby girl awake, while Nathan and big brother Aaron sped behind, all en-route to the nearest children's hospital roughly forty-five minutes away.

In that same radio-thon interview, Brittany explains the day of diagnosis as it unraveled: "As soon as we got there—within the first couple of minutes after I named her symptoms to the E.R. doctor—they said, 'we think she has Type 1 Diabetes'."

Brittany and Nathan were shocked. "I was not expecting that at all. Not in a nine-month-old. I knew the symptoms. I knew people who had it, but in a nine-month-old..."

With that same utter look of disbelief that must have crossed her face at the moment of diagnosis, Brittany explains, "The frequent thirst. The frequent urination. It's something, that you know, you really don't pick up on. She was exclusively breastfed so she was nursing a lot, which is good at that age..." She shrugs her shoulders, "So I didn't think anything of it. And as far as the wet diapers go, it didn't seem anything above ordinary for her, and so it was such a shock."

Brittany and Nathan aren't alone in their failure to recognize the symptoms of the disease. Countless parents have told the story of how they watched symptoms mount before their eyes, only to pass them off as signs of an ordinary bug or a reaction to extreme weather conditions. Down the road, once a diagnosis is given, grief-stricken parents lash out in pain and anger, often blaming each other for their failure to know something was wrong—especially when conflicts over certain parenting decisions already cause tension in the marriage:

"Maybe if you had gotten him vaccinated" one parent might say. Or, "maybe if you were a more involved parent and actually changed a diaper once in a while you would have noticed the problem yourself." The pain a parent feels, thinking that something could have possibly been done sooner had they just been more aware, more knowledgeable, or just a better parent, can be enough to drive anyone to the brink of insanity. At the very least, parents should take comfort in knowing that even medical professionals often overlook the early warning signs.

As Stefany Shaheen recounts in her book "Elle & Coach", a memoir of Stefany's experiences raising a Type-1 adolescent, she had to beg the doctor to do a simple blood-test because he was convinced that Elle did not have diabetes. Stefany's brother-in-law is a type-1 diabetic and she had been doing some research on her daughter's symptoms prior to bringing her to the doctor. She was fairly confident that a blood-test was warranted, but had she not been so persistent, the doctor would have sent them home to further monitor a quickly worsening condition. Fortunately for Elle, Stefany persisted. Unfortunately, not all such stories end happily.

In the early part of 2015, the online community was reeling from news of a little girl named Kycie. As explained on one diabetes-awareness blog, Photograbetic, hosted by a diabetic named Abby, "Kycie's story started on a Monday in January with this precious five-year-old complaining of a tummy ache. Doctors said she had the flu and sent her home. By Friday, she was having seizures and being life-flighted with a correct diagnosis—Type 1 Diabetes." Sadly the realization of what was causing Kycie's symptoms came too late. "Kycie suffered extensive brain damage [from prolonged elevated blood sugars]." The story of her plight flooded newspapers, blogs, and social media sites around the globe. In a memorial tribute article shared by Diabetes.co.uk, Jack Woodfield, a journalist and Type-1 diabetic himself writes, "The Terry family documented Kycie's struggle on Facebook, and the "Kisses for Kycie" page has over 55,000 likes. Not only has brave Kycie inspired the entire diabetes community with her courage, but her story raises awareness of undiagnosed type 1 diabetes."

As many parents will tell, raising awareness is key to battling this disease, and once the initial shock of the diagnosis wears off and they become more comfortable living with their new normal, many families engage themselves in fundraising and diabetes-awareness activities on a regular basis. Organizations like JDRF (the Juvenile Diabetes Research Foundation) continue to push for legislation to make diabetes screenings mandatory, but without an awareness among the primary caregivers—the parents or others who care for children throughout the day—routine screenings are often insufficient when effects of the disease set in between regularly scheduled visits to the doctor. As evidenced by Kycie, it doesn't take long for the symptoms of diabetes to quickly turn disastrous. In some cases missed symptoms or misdiagnoses can mean permanent brain damage or physical disability. In others it can mean death.

Fortunately for the Fenstermakers, the first doctors on the scene were quick to appropriately diagnose young Nora with Type 1. "I had such comfort knowing that right off the bat they knew what it was," says Brittany. "There's a lot of misdiagnosis around Type 1 Diabetes, especially with young kids, and that they knew right away was a great comfort for me."

While Brittany took comfort in knowing that they had gotten Nora the care she needed quickly enough, and that she wouldn't suffer any long-term health effects, the worst was not yet over. Norah was still primarily breastfed at this time. Exclusive breastfeeding at nine-months, while not necessarily common in this country, is a perfectly healthy option for both mothers and babies, and had it not been for the new diagnosis, this mother-baby dyad would have been happy to continue as they were doing. Baby Norah was not yet showing interest in solid foods, and Brittany was happy to continue nourishing her baby in the best way she knew how.

Unfortunately, Norah's new diagnosis meant they might need to make radical changes to the routine—and fast. Breastfeeding can pose a unique challenge for the endocrinology team. Diabetes care relies on careful monitoring of carbohydrate intake and precise insulin calculations, but according to Ann Prentice, and the United Nations University Press, "The composition of breastmilk is not uniform, and the concentrations of many of its constituents change during the lactation period and differ between individual mothers." It is this organic nature of breastmilk to continually adjust to meet the changing needs of the baby that continues to amaze scientists, and foster an entire field of lactation research and management.

It is this same characteristic that causes worry among some endocrinologists. They worry that an inability to definitively calculate the exact carbohydrate intake during any given feeding will make proper care difficult. Fortunately, there is research-based evidence that can help mothers put unnecessary fears to rest. According to that same University Press article, while some components such as protein, fat, micro, and macronutrients may vary a great deal, others such as carbohydrates do not: "Some components show little change, especially those involved in osmoregulation, including lactose [the primary carbohydrate in breastmilk] and sodium." Although there is a difference between early colostrum (in the first week postpartum) and mature milk, it is safe to assume that mature milk consists of 7.5 g per 100 ml (roughly 3.3 oz of milk) or 2.25 grams of carbs per ounce of milk.

With this information in hand, there is only one thing left to determine—the amount of milk consumed during a single nursing session. Since babies take in an average of 5-8 oz of milk per feeding, it is safe to assume that any given nursing session is equivalent to somewhere between 11.25 and 18 grams of carbs (the equivalent of prescribed "between-meal snacks").

Unscientifically speaking (this comes straight from my experience as a mom of four children), pinpointing the exact consumption of a toddler to a narrower window than that is essentially impossible. While we may not be able to measure exactly what comes out of the breast, we at least know that none of the meal was shoved in a diaper or behind the couch for safekeeping. I only wish the same assurances applied to table foods.

For whatever reason though, hospital teams still find comfort in the concept of counting carbs on a plate and all too often urge moms to start moving away from nursing as quickly as possible. As Brittany shares, "Once Norah had a central line put in and IV fluids were started, I asked when I could nurse her. I didn't get a straight answer and I felt paralyzed with fear as I flashed back to our last nursing session. It was hurried. I was trying to get her to breastfeed before we left for the doctor's office, but she really wasn't interested. She had been so unaware of her surroundings at the time and I remember being concerned. It was at this point that I thought, 'What if that was the last time I will ever nurse her again?'" As Brittany looked down at her disconcerted little girl, with wires and tubes strapped to her head, chest and arm, it broke her heart to know that she couldn't offer the one bit of comfort that they both so desperately needed.

As engorgement set in, Brittany set her mind to doing what was needed to make sure that her milk supply wouldn't be compromised and that her milk would be there—in whatever form—for baby Norah when she was ready to have it. Although the conditions were certainly less than ideal (as hours turned to days, dirty laundry was starting to pile up in the corner and the hospital room was starting to take on the feel of an unwelcome hotel room; there was the constant chatter of medical monitors, the pervasive lack of privacy and the never-ending din of medical-talk in the background—stress was at its peak) Brittany requested a pump from the PICU nurse and immediately went to work building a supply in the little hospital refrigerator.

Given the unfavorable conditions and the added strain of watching her precious baby suffer, it's almost miraculous that Britney was able to push through—certainly no one would have blamed her if she hadn't—but in her heart she knew that breastmilk was what was best for her daughter and she was determined to provide it at any cost.

The conversations swirled around her. "This is a very sick little girl..." "Diabetic Ketoacidosis..." "...blood sugar over 600..."

Brittany and Nathan quickly realized that even once Norah's glucose levels were stabilized, managing life with diabetes would be much more difficult than they had originally thought."

"What will we do? How are we going to do this?" they asked each other.

"When will I be able to nurse her again?" Brittany asked the nurse.

"I don't know that you will. For now she is getting everything she needs from the IV," the nurse explained. Brittany's heart sank. Everything is a big word. Sure Norah was getting the fluids, nutrition, and medicine that she needed to stay alive, but was that really everything she needed? Brittany knew she should be relieved that Norah would make a full recovery. She knew that Norah's life should be enough consolation. But it wasn't. Am I being selfish? She thought to herself. "One of the most important parts of our current relationship was being threatened and was on the verge of extinction. I was devastated."

Brittany set to scouring the Internet for answers—just as so many moms who've come before and after have found themselves doing—but to no avail. The truth is, there simply isn't much out there on the subject of nursing diabetic infants and toddlers. Given the relatively small percentage of babies who are still primarily breastfed at this age and present with type 1 diabetes while still nursing, the opportunity (and motivation) for such research is basically nonexistent.

To complicate matters, many members of hospital-based endocrinology teams are ignorant about the benefits of extended breastfeeding even in non-complicated situations—many actually believe that there is no benefit at all beyond young infancy—and easily fall victim to misconceptions regarding the risks of managing diabetes with the imperfect calculations that come along with breastfeeding.

Fortunately for Brittany, social media had something to offer. As Brittany shares in her personal story featured on the well-known KellyMom breastfeeding support site, "I finally stumbled upon a Facebook group for parents of children of type one children. They directed me to the group Diapers and Diabetes, where many other moms continued to breastfeed their type one's after diagnosis. Approval to join the group took a day or two, so I couldn't ask any questions yet, but just knowing there were others brought peace to my soul."

Brittany's words are a poignant reminder of how important it is for mothers of newly diagnosed children to build a strong community of support in those early days—especially in instances when they are attempting to act in accordance with their instincts and find themselves in conflict with standard practice. Parenting a young child with a serious disease can seem isolating, but when parents "follow doctors orders" they at least feel the support of the medical team. When parents challenge standard practice, and question their doctors' methods, they are left to feel that there is no one on their side. In the circumstance of challenging the directive to wean a nursing toddler, mothers often face additional pressure from family members who advise that doctors know best, and that to question them is wrong. This pressure can be especially straining if the mother faces direct opposition from her husband.

Fortunately Nathan was on her side, and as soon as Norah was off the IV, Brittany was permitted to feed her pumped milk from a bottle (providing careful calculations were provided). "It was an emotional moment when I gave her that first bottle of my milk," Brittany shares. "She basically inhaled three bottles worth. My heart was happy and I knew hers was too." The following day Norah was put on an insulin pump (something many babies don't transfer to for months or even years after initial diagnosis). With this new bit of technology, which allows for more fine-tuning of insulin delivery, Brittany was permitted to nurse Norah again directly at the breast. "The ecstasy of that moment was indescribable."

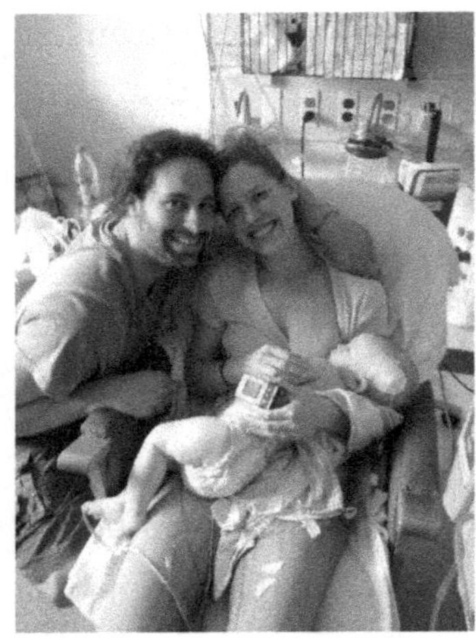

Brittany and her husband Nathan proudly celebrating Norah's return to breast-feeding

Of course, this first post-diagnosis nursing session was just one of the significant triumphs—and struggles—that Brittany and her family would experience together. "After six days in the hospital," Brittany shares on her vlog "Norah's Diabetes Story," we were finally able to head home. We were scared to death and still had so many questions, but we were anxious to have our family together again."

That vlog is just one of Brittany's many accomplishments—and one that makes me cry every time I watch it. Brittany created and posted it within a month of Norah's diagnosis. In the less than two years between that video and her contributing to this book, Brittany and her family have participated in a radio-thon for the hospital where Norah was diagnosed, and multiple walks to raise funds for research and awareness of Type 1 diabetes. Brittany has created a Facebook page that she keeps updated with news of Norah's progress and information on the Type 1 community—Jam for Joy in honor of the family's rock band status. And the family has volunteered their time on numerous occasions to speak out on behalf of JDRF and the ongoing effort to find a cure. Shortly before sharing her story with me, Brittany even took on the challenge of wearing Norah's old glucose monitor for a week so that she could better empathize with her daughter.

Brittany is a strong woman. Not everyone can take on the projects that she and her family have taken on—not doing so certainly doesn't make someone less of a parent. The struggles of caring for a little one with such a temperamental condition is usually work enough in itself! I hope that in sharing this one mother's strength and persistence, I am helping to inspire rather than make anyone feel bad. If it's any consolation, I don't have a vlog, special Facebook page, video documentary, JDRF walk, or band to my name either (even now--9 years after diagnosis). These are all wonderful things that I hope to start getting more involved with in the future, but for now, I often console myself with the knowledge that keeping my child not only alive, but thriving is enough to celebrate in itself.

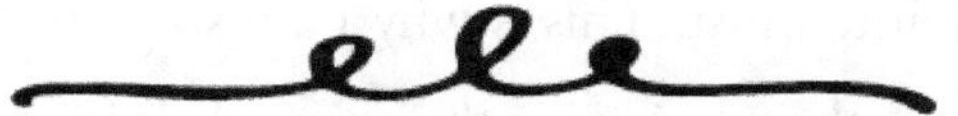

Myra & Weston: Making it Work

To say I'm grateful for online support groups like Diapers and Diabetes is an understatement. Living on a small island makes networking with other Type 1 families a near impossibility (there are only two others that I know of, and both are about a forty-minute drive from my house), and when it comes to managing the day-to-day realities of life with a Type 1 toddler, support is an absolute must. This is why I am so grateful for people like Myra—she is one of the admins for the group, helping to ensure that the conversations stay supportive and the overall tone stays positive.

This is not to say that there isn't quite a bit of venting, virtual crying, and even a bit of swearing here and there (especially from me). None of that is a problem because unloading emotionally is part of what keeps us all sane. At the same time there are certain things that are taboo, such as vaccine debates, and arguments over disease-management styles (such as low-carb vs. standard diets). If left uncontrolled these types of conversations can get wildly out of control with the end result being little more than a bunch of hurt feelings. At one point I remember hearing that a new mom had joined the group only to quit the next day because she came on board at a time when one of these conversations had gotten out of hand. She assumed that being a member would be an added source of stress in her life and quickly opted out. What a terrible loss for us (the group), and her.

That conversation was quickly shut down and deleted, but as most people know, social media networks wield more power than most infectious diseases, capable of spreading hurt and pain in seconds—faster than even the most aggressive cancer. With a current membership of over 1,600 moms—all with different views on parenting, nutrition, and otherwise—there are bound to be conversations that pop up from time to time that step outside the bounds of T1 support, but overall, the space is a wonderful safe-haven for so many of us, and we have people like Myra to thank for keeping it that way.

So in many ways I feel that sharing Myra's own personal story is a great honor. When I spoke with her and learned that her husband was in active military and that she spends many of her days managing this disease as a single parent, the privilege took on even greater significance.

As I learned from Myra, the threat of deployment for her husband hung especially heavy over the household during the winter of 2011-2012. The holiday season had always been crazy for the Murphy family. With the oldest of three sons having his birthday fall smack between Thanksgiving and Christmas, and the fact that they live in the south suburbs of Chicago (aptly named The Windy City for more than a variety of reasons), it has always been just a question of when drama would hit, not if. But this time around, the last days of fall would prove to be the calm before a long and especially stormy season for the Murphys.

With this particular December clocking in as one of the warmest winter months on record—with average high temperatures in the low forties—and a relatively mild and uncharacteristically warm Chicago winter in general about to follow, the weather would prove a stark contrast to the upheaval that would soon change each of their lives forever.

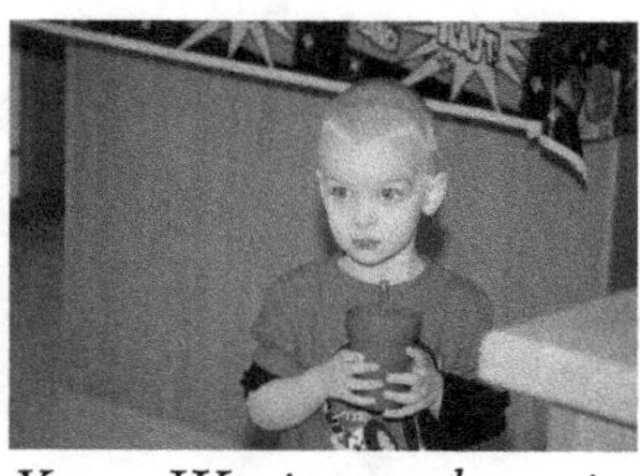

Young Westin, one day prior to diagnosis

December 3 was a Saturday. Myra Murphy spent most of the day busily preparing for her oldest son Hayden's tenth birthday party. There was a good deal of hustle and excitement throughout the house all day long, but by the time the party rolled around, it was fairly obvious that something was drastically wrong with the youngest of the Murphy boys—Weston.

Myra recalls that although Weston had not been himself in a couple of weeks, during the party, things seemed especially off. Kids were running around and playing; eating treats and going wild. "He didn't want any part of any of it," Myra remembers. "He barely ate, and refused pretty much everything but water. He didn't want to play, and spent most of the time passed between his grandmas since I was busy hosting."

Myra, her husband Jordan, and Lorrie—Myra's mom—discussed what to do.

"If he isn't better by Monday we'll bring him to the doctor," Myra said to her mom. "I can take Hayden and Daxton with me tonight" she offered. "This way you can all get some rest."

Lorrie had already suggested that the symptoms seemed characteristic of diabetes, but this wasn't something Myra was open to hearing at the time. "I foolishly told her that babies don't get diabetes," Myra recalls—a dangerous misconception that so many parents hold. Weston, then 2 ½ years old, was still nursing regularly, and co-sleeping with Myra and Jordan, and they felt confident in their ability to keep him safe through the weekend until they could see his regular doctor on Monday.

~ A Note From Erin ~

Though I feel like a bit of a broken record here, I'll point out that nursing beyond a year is less common in this country than others, but a perfectly natural practice. As with the other moms featured in this chapter, Myra is a wonderful example of how extended nursing can fit in with an otherwise typical All-American life. Similarly, Co-sleeping is tradition that is quite common globally, but either less practiced or less talked about in the U.S. It is believed that many parents co-sleep but pretend not to for fear of being judged or criticized by others. While there are safe bed-sharing practices that make this activity a normal and healthy part of parenting, many doctors are quick to discourage parents from sleeping with their children. This encourages the "don't ask don't tell" policy that many parents have with their childrens' pediatricians, limiting the opportunity for open communication on a broad variety of topics.

The best thing a parent can do is connect with a doctor that is supportive of different parenting styles, and respectful of a parents' choices—generally made with their child's best interests in mind. That being said, I live in a small community where medical options are limited. As it is, we have to fly each time we go to see my son's endocrinologist. For parents in similar situations, finding the right fit with a doctor can be a simple matter of luck. In those instances, I highly suggest parents educate themselves on the issues that matter most so that they can participate actively in conversations about their child's care rather than finding themselves being "talked to."

~ End Erin's Note ~

Fortunately, Myra is a strong woman who feels confident enough in her parenting choices to do things as they work for her and her family, rather than worrying about what will make other people happy. Unfortunately, engaging in atypical practices can increase the chances of finger-pointing when things go wrong. For example, one mother was told that nursing her son is what caused his diabetes to go unrecognized and that because of her choice to breastfeed, her child almost died—never mind the fact that the pediatrician had sent the family home twice with a diagnosis of the flu and strict instructions to stay in bed and drink plenty of fluids. Somehow the blame was placed on the mother. Happily, Myra wouldn't have to face the same intimidation and scare tactics when it came to nursing, but her experience regarding the diagnosis was no less traumatic.

"That night I just remember a constant pull during nursing—feeling an almost constant "let down" like he just wasn't getting enough," Myra recalls. "I felt like I didn't sleep at all that night, so when my husband woke up the next morning, he took Weston downstairs with him so I could try to get some sleep."

That break only lasted about twenty minutes and would be the last rest Myra would see for quite a while.

"Hurry up, Myra. Get dressed."

In her stupor, Myra tried to make sense of what was going on. Jordan explained, "I gave Weston a bottle of Gatorade and he chugged the whole thing down, but then immediately threw it all up. I Googled the symptoms and the first 100 results that came back were just for Type 1 Diabetes. I think—"

She stopped him. She didn't want to hear the words that would make her worst nightmare come true. "We took two of the fastest showers ever and rushed to our local urgent care," Myra remembers. "It was a first-come, first-served type of place. When we pulled into the parking lot, another car pulled in behind us and raced into the handicap spot so the daughter could get in and sign in before us." Myra was livid.

By the time Myra and Jordan parked and got into the office there was a line of four families in front of them, including the girl and her mom. Myra bit her tongue and did everything to keep all of her emotions in check. "I held my baby in my arms as each person was called before us and just watched him fade right before my eyes. The wait seemed endless, but we finally got called back to Triage."

Jordan explained to the intake nurse, "We think he has Type 1 Diabetes."

Looking at his listless body the nurse asked, "Is it possible he has a head injury?" She tried to stand him up and place him on the scale for a weight check, but in his fragile state, he couldn't support the weight of his own body. Realizing the urgency of the situation, the nurse transferred the family into an exam room to wait for a doctor.

As the doctor walked into the room, Jordan urged again, "We think he has Type 1 Diabetes. Please..."

The doctor immediately called for a lab technician to bring a glucose monitor. "It was a huge meter," Myra recalls. "Within seconds the results were in: HI. I knew what that meant. Our baby had diabetes."

Myra was savvier than many parents at this stage. For many who have never even seen a glucometer, the letters and numbers flashing across the monitor are generally meaningless. Of course making sense of the readout is a skill that parents of Type 1 children have to learn all too intimately.

~ A Note From Erin ~

Because those whose life revolves around managing a chronic illness are always looking for a way to make light of challenging situations, the abbreviated version of "high"—HI—that appears on monitors has become a common source of merry-making on support boards. Posts to the effect of "Why is my monitor always mocking me with that cheery 'HI'?" reflect the ongoing challenges of diabetics and their caregivers to keep blood glucose levels in a safe ranges.

Most handheld glucometers have the ability to read blood glucose levels between roughly 45 mg/dL (2.5 mmol/L outside of the US) at the low end and 500 mg/dL (27.7 mmol/L outside of the US) at the high end. Some of the newer models will have a slightly broader range from 20 mg/dL (roughly 1.1 mmol/L) to 600 mg/dL (33.3 mmol/L). While even some numbers within this range (45-65 on the low end and 250-500 on the high end) are considered abnormal and can cause long-term consequences if unchecked for periods of time, numbers that are too low or high to register are extremely dangerous and register simply as "LOW" or "HI" indicating a need for immediate attention. In order for doctors to get a more accurate picture of what the numbers might be, blood has to be drawn and sent to the lab for analysis.

~ End Erin's Note ~

Like so many other young children when they are first diagnosed, Weston's numbers were too far out of range for the doctor's glucometer to calculate a numeric reading.

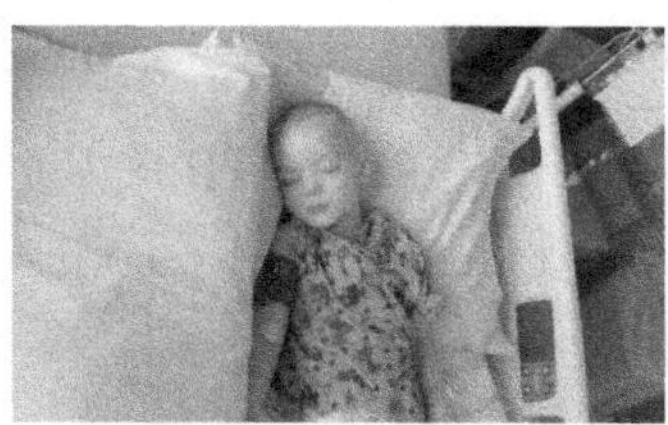
Westin in the hospital, shortly after admission

"He is severely dehydrated," the doctor explained, "We need to start an IV."

"I don't understand," questioned Myra. "He nursed all night long!"

The doctor pulled the skin away on Weston's small lifeless hand, and it just stayed that way—it didn't bounce back like skin normally does—"That's a sign of extreme dehydration," the doctor explained."

The nurse tried to start the IV, but couldn't find a vein. "I'll be right back..." the doctor promised as he hurried out of the room.

A minute later he was back to report that they would be transporting Weston immediately to the hospital.

"Should we get him dressed?" Myra asked.

"No," he explained. "I've already called the ambulance and they'll be here any minute. You need to go immediately."

The paramedics rushed into the room and placed Weston on a gurney.

"You can ride with him in the ambulance," they said the Myra. Jordan would be left to drive himself to the hospital.

"They strapped us into the gurney," Myra recalls, "with me slightly propped up and him on my chest. I covered both of us with my coat. Then we were off.

"I just remember looking out at the traffic behind us through the little window at the back of the ambulance. There was a section of road construction on the way to the hospital, but since it was Sunday morning, there were no construction workers and the ambulance was able to speed through the construction zone. I watched all the cars fall away so fast as we raced ahead."

In the time it took the paramedics to get Myra and Weston settled for the drive, Jordan had rushed ahead and wound up arriving at the hospital before them. He was there to meet the ambulance as it pulled up to the emergency entrance and ran along with Myra and the emergency responders as they whisked baby Weston into the ER.

Although Weston was quickly deteriorating, fading in and out of consciousness, Myra and Jordan quickly found—as many parents in this situation have—that even an incredibly sick child will fight to the death to avoid being stuck by needles. "They held us in the emergency ward for several hours trying to get blood," Myra remembers. "Weston still had enough fight left in him that it took four people, including my big strong husband to hold him down to try to get the blood from his tiny body."

Hours passed, and eventually they were transferred to the Pediatric Intensive Care Unit, or PICU—what would become their home for the remainder of their hospital stay. The room was small, with little room beyond Weston's bed and his accompanying medical equipment.

"Fortunately he was old enough to get a regular bed that I could sleep in with him each night," Myra says, "Otherwise there would have been no place for me to stay."

Between the sense of confinement and the constant influx of doctors and nurses, it was difficult for Myra to settle her nerves. One nurse in particular checked in on them every fifteen minutes on the dot. Myra assumed that things were slow, and that the nurse was just being friendly, but as she later learned, the 15-minute checks were mandatory—Weston was the sickest child in the ward.

"They told us he was in DKA" Myra explains, and that they needed to bring his blood sugar down, but slowly.

"The insulin is taking effect a bit more quickly than we'd like" the doctor explained, "and his blood sugar is dropping too quickly. We need him to drink some juice."

But again, Weston's spunk kicked in and he refused.

"Can I nurse him?" Myra asked.

The doctor was hesitant at first, not knowing how to account for the carbohydrates in breast milk, but he knew Weston needed something quickly and agreed to let Myra give nursing a try. Her milk worked to bring Weston's glucose levels back up to a more comfortable level (much to everyone's great relief), and in time a nurse returned with some great news—she was able to get an approximate carb count (likely from someone in labor and delivery) so that nursing could be continued and the carbohydrates in Myra's breast milk could be accurately factored into Weston's management plan.

"We got so lucky with our endo team" Myra points out. "Anytime an issue came up, Martha, our nurse practitioner just kind of shrugged her shoulders and said, 'We'll make it work'—and they did."

~ A Note From Erin ~

Myra knows she was lucky because she has heard from too many other mothers who have been urged to wean. Because the breakdown of nutrients in breast milk isn't as standardized as that of commercial cow's milk, doctors and nurses are quick to suggest an immediate shift to table foods or formula, which they feel can be more accurately measured. What most don't realize is that while certain components vary from day to day, or even hour to hour, others (such as carbohydrates) are actually quite consistent, allowing for reliable estimates to be made. For a child over the age of 6 months, who consumes roughly 5-8 ounces of milk per feeding, the average carbohydrate intake averages roughly 15 grams—consistent with the guidelines for between-meal "snacks" for children with diabetes.

Unfortunately, endocrinology is a highly specialized field, with doctors and nurses required to stay on top of overwhelming amounts of knowledge specific to their area of expertise—breastfeeding science is generally something that does not fit into that tremendous scope of study. As a result, many working on the endocrinology team are ignorant about the benefits of breastfeeding, the risks of abrupt weaning, and the compatibility of continued nursing with diabetes management. As a result, most moms report "being bullied" into weaning because taking the baby off breast milk is the easier option for the medical staff.

~ End Erin's Note ~

At one point, when asked whether or not she wished they had been transferred to the children's hospital in Chicago rather than staying in the small suburban hospital by their home, she said, "I'm actually glad it worked out the way it did because it seems like a lot of children's hospitals are very rigid with their management plans. I felt like our endo really understood that each child is unique and didn't try to fit us into the diabetes box." Based on the stories shared by countless other mothers in regard to their inability to continue comfortably nursing their newly diagnosed child while in the hospital, it seems that Myra might be quite right about how lucky they were to avoid a transfer.

And so they remained—in the regular ward of a somewhat rural hospital, far away from highly modernized, brightly decorated Children's Hospital of midtown Chicago. As Myra lay on that little hospital bed she would share with Weston each night, relieved that she could finally comfort him the way that felt most natural to them both, she finally was able to get some rest. She lay there, just holding him, as their first long day came to an end.

As December 5, the second day of their new lives, set in, Weston started showing signs of improvement. His spirits were picking up and he was more communicative. But only so much peace was to be had. The frequent blood draws continued, and each time the nurses approached to take their required sample, Weston would cry, "No Mommy!" It was too much for Myra to bear.

"At one point I ran out of the room in tears unable to watch everything they were doing to my baby," Myra remembers.

The hours were long, but things seemed to be moving in the right direction. By the end of that day, Weston was able to transition from an insulin drip to the shots that Myra and Jordan would soon learn to administer on their own. They were finally moved from the cramped spaces of the PICU to a regular room in the pediatric ward. Weston ate his first solid meal in days, and big brothers Hayden and Daxton were able to sneak in for a short visit. The boys' excitement to see their parents and brother was contagious, and their visit helped lift everyone's spirits.

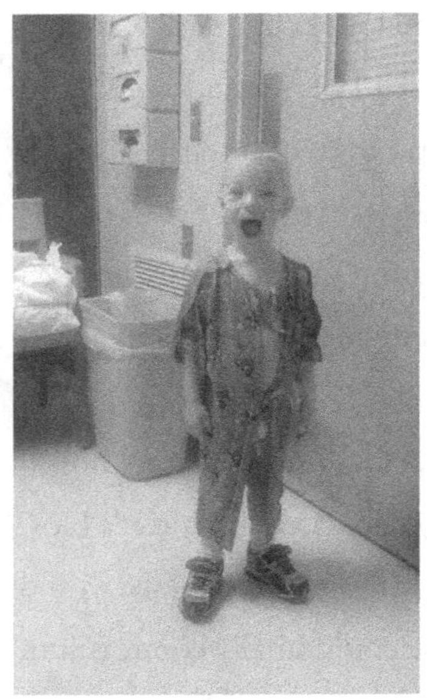

Westin's spirits start to lift as insulin begins to do its job and the family nears discharge.

December 6 marked their third day in the hospital and the official start of Diabetes Management Bootcamp. First Myra and Jordan practiced drawing up syringes and tapping carefully with their fingernails to release the tiny little bubbles that can have a huge impact when trying to measure such small doses of insulin. A few bubbles can mean the difference between ½ unit and 1 full unit—a big difference to a child Weston's size. So they continued to practice.

Eventually the time came for real-life training. Jordan first injected Myra with a syringe of saline solution. "I was surprised by how much it stung!" she recalls.

Finally the real practice would start, in the only way it could, on little Weston. And while it was difficult for all of them to get used to their new roles as patient and care takers, they were able to manage and eventually discharged to continue their learning at home.

December 7 marked their first day home from the hospital. To mark the occasion, Myra updated her Facebook status: "WE ARE HOME!!!! HOLY SH*T – now we really have to do it all! Getting ready to surprise my big boys when they get off the school bus."

This was soon followed by her self-congratulatory (rightfully so) post: "We kept Weston alive all night & only had to call nurse Martha once. Yay Us!!"

Elements of normalcy started to creep back into their lives as they fell back into their regular routines—bus drop-offs and pick-ups, meal preparation and cleanups, and good-night kisses as each boy peacefully rested a head on his own pillow for the night; each grateful to be comfortably resting in his own bed.

On December 9, Myra posted, "The boys just all gave me a good laugh when they stripped down to their underwear (and Weston in his diaper) so they could dance to "Sexy and I know it." While so much had changed in a short time, the Murphys were learning that real life would carry on—despite the finger sticks, midnight checks, and intermittent tears that each would shed for the loss of the way things used to be.

On December 14 Myra took Weston to the doctor for his first check since being released from the hospital. He was so traumatized by everyone in scrubs, and Myra quickly realized that the real recovery was only just beginning.

With the threat of deployment still hanging over their heads, some days seemed longer than others, but Christmas proved to be merry and bright, serving as a welcome distraction to the events in the days of Advent. As if a gift from Santa Claus himself, the Chicagoland weather was especially beautiful on that Christmas Day and all were grateful to celebrate with a bar-b-qued feast of high-protein grilled steaks, and a few carbohydrate-dense, but carefully counted potatoes.

Footnote for Myra's Story

Breastmilk Information and statistics come from Ann Prentice

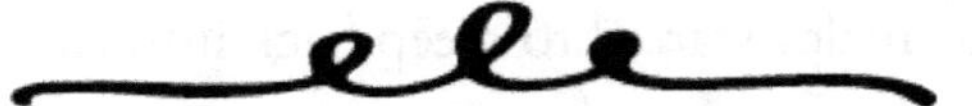

Wendy & Liam: The Early Days

When I first started putting this project together, I was determined to balance the chapters (whatever that meant to me at the time). I connected with so many wonderful women and would have loved to have shared all of their stories, but this chapter on "Breastfeeding at Diagnosis" was becoming a bit top-heavy and I felt the need to move on to other chapters. It is now 2022—8 years after I initially started interviewing mothers and sorting their stories into chapters. Wendy was one of the first women to reach out, but because I already had 3 stories about mothers' struggles to continue breastfeeding past diagnosis, I put her narrative to the side.

Fortunately, Wendy and I have managed to keep in touch over the years, as she has gleefully and graciously updated me on her pregnancy with and the birth of Liam's younger sister Ella. When it finally came time to revitalize this project, I posted a call for submissions in one of the groups that Wendy and I share in common, and she again volunteered to contribute her story.

Most of what I will share about Wendy and Liam will be found in Chapter 5, as I do my best to capture what an amazing woman Wendy is in managing all of Liam's multiple conditions, while also giving so much love and personalized attention to her younger daughter Ella. But as I read back through everything that Wendy shared with me throughout the years, I couldn't bring myself to discard the story of her breastfeeding journey with Liam. What follows below is the heroic and inspiring story of a woman who pushed through countless medical obstacles to provide her son with what she knew to be the gift of love and life.

Wendy initially reached out to me through Facebook Messenger in April 2017 and shared the following with me:

Hi Erin! My son Liam has brain abnormalities, global delay, seizure disorder, profound hearing loss in his right ear, a g-tube, gastroparesis and T1D. He has so many things going on that it can make your head spin. We go to regular therapies every week and a special neuroplasticity therapy monthly as well as many many doctors appointments for his various conditions. We don't have his underlying diagnosis yet. We are awaiting results from extensive genetic testing. He was Dx T1 in September and we have been on the Omnipod for about 1.5-2 months now. We also got on Dexcom about a month after diagnosis.

As I explained to her at the time, I was a bit awe-struck that she would even reach out to me. I knew how much difficulty I was having with meeting all of Connor's needs, but that seemed to pale in comparison to what Wendy was managing. And here she was offering to take the time to share her story with others. When I said all of this to her, she responded, "I really want to be able to help others as much as I can [to] navigate what can be absolutely crazy, confusing and frustrating." Of course, this is similar to what every woman who has participated in this project has said to me. Nancy, who you'll meet in Chapter 5, explains how finding others' stories through podcasts and online support groups was a literal lifeline for her and how she wanted to be able to offer that same gift forward by sharing her story through this project.

Hearing Nancy's words and reading back through Wendy's Facebook messages to me over the years, has reminded me of how important it is to get these stories out there. This project has become bigger than anything I could have created on my own. And as I read through Wendy's 5-year-old message, explaining to me that she was communicating with me while hooked up to a TENS machine, trying to undo the damage of constantly carrying around a 30 lb toddler, with multiple delays, along with his 50 lb.

wheelchair in and out of the car on a daily basis, I am reminded of the utter selflessness of the women who have contributed to this book.

During that time of early written correspondence with Wendy, Liam was 3 years old and still nursing and co-sleeping. He was also one year into his diabetes diagnosis. She told me then, "Really, considering everything, he is doing amazing. He looks terrible on paper and it is extremely hard, but he is making progress." I can't think of a single sentence to capture Wendy's essence better than that one right there. One thing I've noticed about Wendy over the years is that she truly finds joy in her son's milestones—however big or small. She captures him in wonderfully joyful pictures as he is truly living and loving life. In one image, they're in a big field and Liam is being swung around by his dad, as sister Ella jumps up and down in the background, cheering them on. It is a picture of the "normalcy" that we all work so hard to hold onto when the rough days try to drag us down. If I had to guess, I would assume that Wendy would tell anyone reading this book that the secret to managing life with a child with disabilities is to celebrate every positive moment when it comes along.

When we first started trying to collaborate on her story, she apologized for stepping back from the work and explained that Liam had had over 1,000 seizures in the span of 2 days. I responded "Please don't worry about me. This book is a long work in progress because our lives always take priority." Little did I know at the time how long the project would take, but I'm glad the delays allowed me to bring Wendy back into the fold. She told me that she knew she had to prioritize Liam's needs but that she also really wanted to contribute because she felt it would be both helpful to others and cathartic for her. And that was the last we communicated for nearly a year.

When I heard back from her next, it was June of 2018 and Wendy was starting to undergo fertility treatments. She was reaching out to see if it was safe for her to continue breastfeeding. Although we went back and forth about breastfeeding while trying to conceive through IVF, what struck me most was that she and Liam were still in a nursing relationship, despite all the pushback she received from doctors in the early days following Liam's diagnosis.

In August of 2018, she reached out to let me know that she had successfully conceived and was 8 weeks along with a new baby. She was facing pushback again, but this time because a nurse in one of her online breastfeeding groups had "ratted her out" to the doctor for nursing while pregnant. The doctor confirmed that Wendy's pregnancy hormones were in the normal range but reiterated that weaning was still her best choice. Liam was 4 by this time and Wendy felt confident that the intermittent "comfort nursing" that he was doing wouldn't pose a risk to her unborn child. Considering all that she was managing with Liam, it saddens me to think about how much pushback she got from doctors who tried to convince her to stop nursing him.

Throughout that year of pregnancy, Wendy continued to share pictures and updates with me about how continued nursing sessions were going. In one message she wrote, "I wanted to share this with you in case you have any way of getting this hold into any literature for LC's [lactation consultants]." She shared some pictures with me and explained that she was using a hold that she had figured out on her own to support her son's head, which still greatly lacked muscle control.

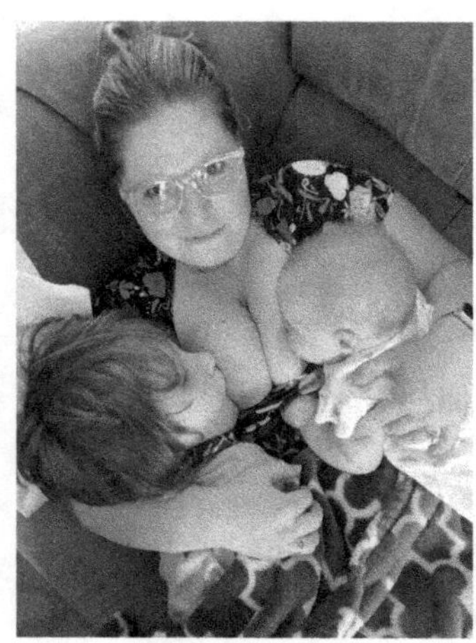

June, 2019: Wendy messaged me this picture with a note that read, "Check out what I managed the other day! Most successful tandem session so far."

She told me, "I provide support behind the head with my arm and I use my pointer finger for cheek support while using the thumb, middle and ring fingers to provide breast support and breast compressions. Generally this does best in a side lying type of position." This was Wendy again, trying to make sure that anything she had learned from her own experiences and that could possibly be used to help others, would have a chance of getting out into the world. Finally, in March of 2019, she shared a glowing picture of herself tandem nursing Liam and his newborn sister Ella for the first time.

Wendy's breastfeeding journey is certainly unlike most others, but it's such a wonderful testament to what can be accomplished with the right combination of confidence and determination.

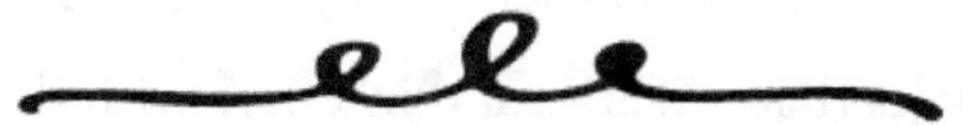

Jessica & Oliver: Advocating for the Needs of the Nursing Toddler

Jessica wrote to me, "I felt like my body was failing me the more I saw him drinking bottles constantly." Oliver was still nursing in the months leading up to diagnosis, and as he continued to lose weight, while demanding bottles to supplement what Jessica could provide at the breast, it led her to conclude that her body just couldn't produce enough milk to meet his needs. "It broke my heart. It broke me down. I felt so inadequate. I felt like I was failing him! I had postpartum depression after I had him so all I was doing was blaming myself. I lost faith in my body as his body was failing him."

~ A Note From Erin ~

As a lactation consultant, I've seen far too many women define the quality of their mothering by their success or "failure" with nursing their child. While the fact that humans, like all mammals, have the wonderful ability to nourish their young with their milk, there are countless obstacles that can arise and interfere with that process, and when a mother hits a breastfeeding obstacle that she can't overcome, it can lead to profound grief. Although some of the obstacles many women face today are the result of living in an increasingly technological world and the changes in societal norms that separate mother and child earlier and earlier in the postpartum period, breastfeeding challenges are not unique to the modern world.

~ Continued Note ~

Before the advent of formula, mothers who ran into challenges with nursing their babies could turn to other lactating women in the community for support. Even in the mid-20th century, after formula started to grow in popularity, the sharing of breastmilk was recognized as a safe and healthy practice without the stigma of failure that so many women feel today when they are unable to provide their babies with sufficient human milk. My own mother was part of a milk-sharing community when I was an infant, and she has shared stories with me about how she and other lactating women would take turns breastfeeding another woman's baby in the community—and that was in the 1970s. Although milk-banks and the milk-sharing process has grown in sophistication in recent decades, sharing milk is not exactly a common practice in America, and women who find themselves unable to nurse their child to the point of cherub are often wracked with guilt.

~ End Erin's Note ~

As Jessica explains, that guilt can often result in clinical depression. "The days leading up to my son's diagnosis are a blur but crystal clear at the same time," Jessica explains. "I kept thinking that he looked like he had lost a lot of weight. He looked so skinny. I had begun to doubt my body's ability to produce enough milk for him. He was nursing non-stop and taking at least 2 bottles a day on top of that. I shouldn't have been as upset as I was about it—he was 16 months old after all." But what we should feel as mothers and what we do feel as mothers are often quite different.

Jessica started to find ways to justify the sudden weight-loss and increased appetite. "He was skinny because he was running more...He was drinking bottles because he was so busy and getting ready to wean..." But of course what Jessica didn't know was that something very different than typical growth and development was at play here. Oliver wasn't losing weight because "he was running more," just as Connor wasn't constantly getting sick because it was "cold and flu season." but as far too many of us parents of the youngest diabetics come to learn, Type 1 does not present in young children the way it does in adolescents and older individuals. The chronic thirst that some consider to be a tell-tale sign in older children looks more like hunger in children who are still primarily on liquid diets. And the frequent urination that is so obvious in the school-aged child can be easy to overlook when diapers are still involved.

For Jessica, all of this was even more confusing because she was still nursing her 3-year-old, who was absolutely thriving on mother's milk. As she says, her inability to keep up with Oliver's nutritional needs was just so foreign to her. And the more she thought about it, the sadder she became.

In the two days leading up to their inevitable visit to the emergency room, Oliver started acting very lethargic. Just as I did with Connor, Jessica brushed it off as a bug and held a bit of a nurse-in, providing extra skin-to-skin contact and love. At the risk of sounding cliche, if I had a dollar for every mother who tried to love her child through that pre-diabetic stage, I'd most certainly be driving a much nicer car than I do now! But as we've all come to realize, love alone is no match for an undiagnosed auto-immune disease.

Twenty-four hours into her nurse-in, Jessica called the pediatrician. Things were going from bad to worse. By the time they got to the doctor's office, all Oliver wanted to do was lay on the cold tile floor. This actually gave Jessica cause to chuckle—it's much easier to see your child as silly rather than painfully sick. In the days and months that followed, Jessica would think back on this moment in "absolute horror," guilt-ridden by the fact that she had laughed while her son suffered at her side. But, of course, she had no way of knowing his pain. None of us did. But that's ok; we'll torture ourselves over this lack of knowing anyway—because anger is a natural part of grief.

As Jessica thinks back to that fateful day, she recalls how "his tiny body was slowly turning into a lifeless rag doll that cried for mama constantly." He had lost 7 pounds in 6 months, weighing in at just 21 pounds at 16 months old. "But, for whatever reason, this was not alarming to [Oliver's doctor] in the least." The pediatrician suggested that it was probably just a virus and instructed Jessica to give Oliver ibuprofen or Tylenol and to only take him to the ER if his fever went up over 103—instructions that quite literally could have cost Oliver his life.

For Oliver, it is fortunate that his mother trusted her instincts over the advice of the pediatrician. Although they left the doctor's office temporarily relieved that Oliver's lethargy was probably due to nothing more than a common bug, Jessica soon realized that something more serious was going on. Even though diabetes was the furthest thing from her mind (she thought Oliver might be suffering from meningitis), she knew that he needed urgent medical care. And so 12 hours later, at 1 in the morning, she made the life-saving decision to take her son to the ER.

~ A Note From Erin ~

Unfortunately, far too many pediatricians are unskilled in recognizing the early warning signs of Diabetic Ketoacidosis (DKA) in young children. This is the phase in disease progression where the body literally starts to break down, as fat stores are used for energy in the absence of insulin. While it is not typically my practice to criticize the medical community (there are multiple medical professionals in our family and I have the highest respect for all of them), it is all too common for parents to share stories of dismissive doctors sending home children in DKA when they should be sending them to the emergency room. I'm not sure why this is still so commonplace, when it is easy enough to make blood-sugar screenings part of routine medical evaluations, but I guess if there is any silver-lining to be found here, it is that parents should easily be able to absolve themselves of guilt for "missing the signs" when medical professionals do it every day.

~ End Erin's Note ~

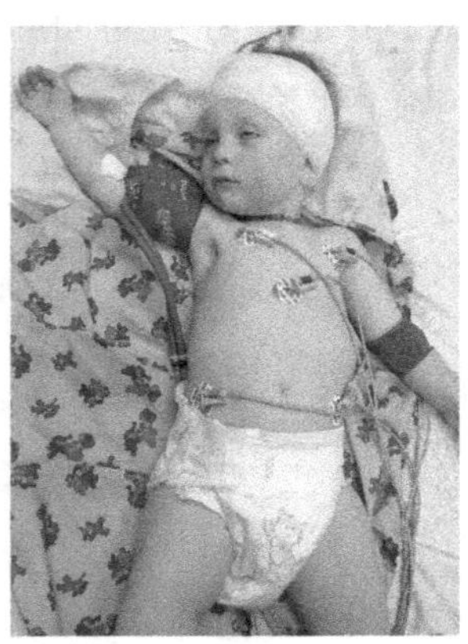

Oliver in the hospital in the hours immediately following diagnosis

The emergency room staff instantly recognized the urgency of Oliver's situation. As Jessica vividly recalls, "They did a full work up—and my boy...my active, crazy, climbing-on-everything little boy, laid there as lifeless as could be."

Jessica tried to nurse Oliver, but he could barely latch onto the breast at that point. "I remember how dry his mouth was—His tongue felt like sandpaper and he couldn't latch" she says. Although he wasn't truly transferring milk, Jessica cradled him at the breast, knowing that it was the only small comfort she could offer him in that moment.

"I was devastated. I remember the moment the doctor came back and said 'diabetes'. That was the only word I can remember coming out of her mouth."--That shared moment of truth that we all remember so well.

"The room was spinning. Everyone was moving so fast. A crash cart was moved into the room. I didn't realize it then, but they all thought my baby boy wasn't going to make it."

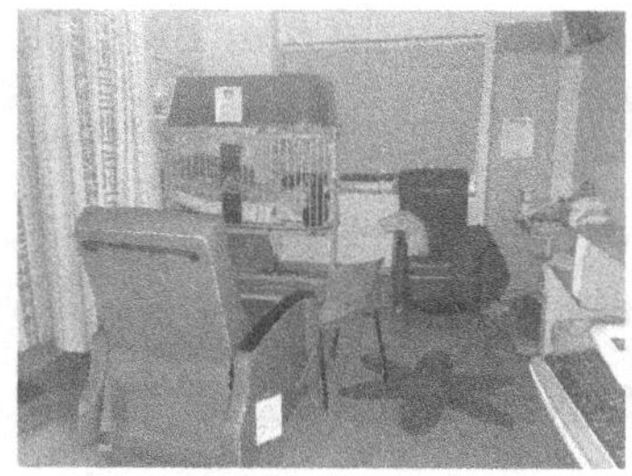

Oliver's hospital "cage" as Jessica refers to it.

It is impossible to communicate to anyone—unless they've been there themselves—what it feels like to watch your child slip away from you. To think that your child is going to die before your eyes. You want to think, "This can't be real. This can't be happening." But it is. And no matter how much time passes, that moment is one that you carry with you always. As the "diaversaries" pass, and you take joy in knowing how far you've both come, those twinges of pain (and guilt) will pop up every now and again. You'll remember how close you came to a different reality. You'll fault yourself for not doing a better job—both in the early days, and as growth spurts and life changes make disease management feel more like a reality show than real life.

As Jessica points out, it is impossible to understand the full scope of what a diagnosis of diabetes means in those early days. Even as the weeks pass, it is impossible to foresee the challenges that this disease will throw your way. In those first days following diagnosis, Jessica kept trying to get people to acknowledge that by trusting her instincts, she had saved her son's life. That if she had followed the pediatrician's instructions and waited it out longer, her son would be dead.

It's a strange thing for a mother to wish for—an acknowledgement that her child was miraculously saved from the grips of death. But I can understand the desire. In those early days, such an acknowledgement is a gift. Like a badge that says, "You cracked the code. You have the power within you." Because that's what we're all wondering as we first process the news. "Can I do this?" And yes, as we all eventually come to learn, we can. And do. Repeatedly.

Following the initial ambulance ride and hospital transfer, Jessica and Oliver were set up in a room in the PICU. It was 6 am by the time they got settled into their new quarters and Jessica was running on pure adrenaline. When Oliver had first arrived at the hospital, his blood sugar was so high that even the advanced meters couldn't register a reading. Finally, a good 24-hours later, after receiving some insulin, Oliver's numbers started to drop. They had a reading for the first time—1472. Even for those of us who have found ourselves, with child in arms, knocking at death's door, this is a staggering number.

Jessica also points out that although she didn't understand the significance at the time, Oliver's pH was 7.1. With the normal range being anywhere from 7.35—7.45, this number might not seem startling at first, but a brief Google search suggests that a pH reading just slightly lower than Oliver's on that day (6.8) is considered "incompatible with life." Now that Jessica is a registered nurse and understands how critical pH balance is to human function, she says it "blows her mind" to think of the truly critical nature of her son's condition at that time.

Unfortunately, obtaining these numbers was only the beginning. The "delicate and dangerous game," as Jessica describes it, of balancing his numbers is a tedious process and is quite overwhelming for parents without a medical background.

~ A Note From Erin ~

Parents start the process of learning how to check blood sugar and give corrections while in the hospital, but it can take many months for insulin needs to level out. And of course, that leveling is only temporary at best. As time passes, the "honeymoon phase" will eventually come to an end. The pancreas will no longer provide intermittent drips of insulin and dosing ratios will change. And as children continue to grow, their needs will continue to change. Eventually, the family will come to find its "new normal," but during that initial hospital stay, the desperate need for a return to normalcy is gut-wrenching.

~ End Erin's Note ~

As Jessica explains, it was 4 days before she was allowed to nurse Oliver again. She says that she uses the term (allowed) loosely. I don't. I remember how adamant the PICU staff was that I abstain from all nursing. Determination be damned—they sure can put the fear of God into you! So, Jessica pumped every 2-3 hours (both to maintain her supply and to create a reserve of breastmilk). Fortunately for her, one of her best friends is a lactation consultant, so she had an advocate in her corner. But even I, a lactation consultant myself, had a difficult time convincing the PICU staff that a return to breastfeeding was not only safe, but critical for the emotional well-being of both me and my son.

As Jessica shares, all of the doctors were focused on carb counting and how breastmilk would need to be fed through a bottle for an accurate count. But, of course, breastfeeding is about so much more than carbs and calories, and Jessica knew that. She knew that breastfeeding was the one bit of normalcy that she could offer her son (and herself) and she was committed to finding her way back—regardless of the warnings that she would just be making her life more difficult.

Whenever she picked Oliver up, she became more convinced that there had to be a way to make it work. He kept pointing to her breasts and asking to nurse. Telling him 'no' was just devastating to them both. It eventually got so bad, that she couldn't even hold him. Being in his mother's arms without being able to nurse was so upsetting to him that holding him started to feel like punishment. "Oliver spent days in a crib that looked like a jail," Jessica recalls painfully. "He was almost lifeless in there. He was either sleeping or crying out for me. It was too much to bear. I found myself needing to walk away."

The doctors continued to push pumping and bottles on Jessica. The grief was overwhelming, and she found herself starting to fall apart. There had to be a way.

Eventually, she found her inner warrior. She knew she needed to stand up for her son. She knew that a return to breastfeeding was the one way she could help them both start to heal from the trauma.

When Oliver was finally allowed to eat food again, she initially gave him a bottle. He only drank 2 ounces of her milk, but it was a start. Shortly after, they were transferred out of the PICU and into a regular room. She found herself confronted with the same anti-breastfeeding mentality that she had been up against in the PICU, but eventually met a compassionate nurse who was willing to help her on her crusade.

They agreed to carefully monitor Oliver's blood sugar throughout the night so that Jessica could reintroduce him to the breast. Oliver latched on instantly. Jessica describes the dramatic change that followed: "It was like a different child was in my arms. Not the one I had seen for the past few days. Not the child I had to walk away from. This was MY baby. And my baby suckled happily on and off for the next hour or so with little to no changes in his blood sugar. It was amazing! I cried tears of relief. Oliver slept so comfortably and happily on my chest that night."

Unfortunately, the doctors started pushing her to bottle-feed again the next day. But as Jessica explains, Oliver knew better. Just as his mother had found her warrior, so too had he. He refused all bottles entirely.

From that point on, Jessica chose her battles carefully. She "just started to do the nod and agree" thing when doctors tried to convince her that bottle-feeding would be best for them long-term. While it is understandable that doctors want to control as much as possible, there are just some things that are best left to nature--or at the very least, appreciated as natural and accommodated as such.

"Words cannot describe the difference I saw in my son when he was finally able to nurse again," Jessica explained. "It was night and day. You could see the anguish and pain on his face every time I had to tell him no. I could see the disconnect. I could see how heartbroken and confused he was. The moment I let him finally breastfeed again, it was like all of that was gone. Despite being hooked up to machines and being poked and prodded at constantly, everything was alright with the world. Finally, being able to breastfeed brought my son--the one I had known--back to me. I am forever grateful to the nurse who helped me achieve this. For my friends who supported me. And for myself, for always fighting for what he needs. I can't tell you how much seeing our breastfeeding relationship renew itself like this has restored my faith in my own body as well," Jessica shared.

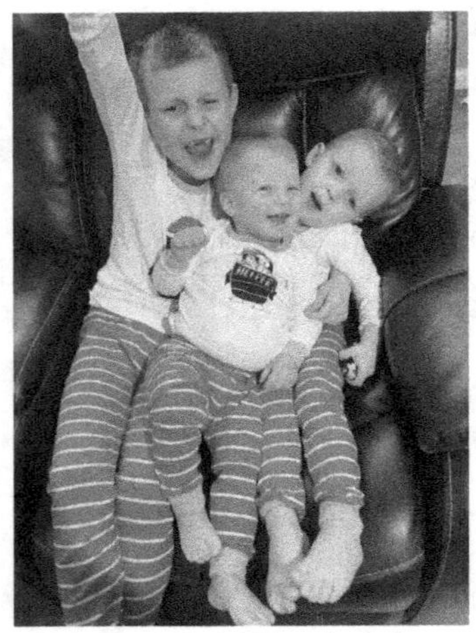

Oliver with his big brothers on his first day home from the hospital

Jessica's words are both heart-warming and frustrating. While it is reassuring to know that Jessica eventually triumphed and she and Oliver were able to reclaim their breastfeeding relationship, it is disheartening to know that like Jessica, so many mothers and nurslings are still suffering through type of trauma on a regular basis.

And sometimes the push-back doesn't end when the family walks, for the last time, through the hospital doors. "Occasionally, I still get slack from the endocrinologist's office," Jessica lamented. The latest struggle was over a battle with high blood sugars and ketones.

"And if only I wasn't breastfeeding, we wouldn't have ended up in the ER' after fighting with it for 2 days." As Jessica points out, this is the kind of thinking that needs to change.

And on this note, I think it best to let Jessica have the last word on the importance of establishing a collaborative relationship with the endocrinology team:

"If I was the kind of person who let others tell me what to do...if I was the kind of mother who blindly listened to every doctor--we would have weaned. Heck, if I had listened to my pediatrician, my son would be dead. What T1 mothers need are doctors who listen to us. Doctors who can meet us where we are. Yes, managing type 1 diabetes in a toddler is tough. And maybe you think breastfeeding is a curve ball. But you figure it out. You make it work. Because it's not just about the milk. It's the relationship that has been built between mother and child, and it needs to be nurtured through such a taxing disease. I know at the end of the day, no matter how exhausted [my] T1 has got me, I know that I will get to sit down and cuddle my sweet boy and nurse him, and connect with him before putting him to bed."

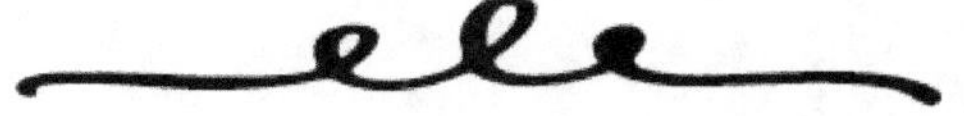

Chapter Four

Changing Family Dynamics

The stories in this chapter illustrate the myriad of ways life can change after a young child is diagnosed with a chronic disease. Roughly 50% of marriages in the U.S. end in divorce—most people are well aware of this statistic. Unfortunately, divorce rates are significantly higher in families with a child who lives with a lifetime medical condition—the rates are actually closer to 75%. And the risk of divorce is only one of the potential challenges that newly diagnosed T1 families face.

Whereas some families might be complete by the time a child is diagnosed—the parents not intending to have another baby despite the current health status of their children—others are only just getting started. When parents find themselves grappling with a new diagnosis in one child just as they were preparing to try for another one (or, in some cases, unexpectedly surprised by a new pending arrival), the fear and guilt they feel can be overwhelming. Mothers worry about their ability to manage the typical exhaustion of pregnancy coupled with round-the-clock monitoring of their young diabetic child. And parents deal with overwhelming feelings of guilt that they may be bringing a child into the world who is more likely than average to be plagued by the same disease.

In other instances, multiple family members are diagnosed within a relatively short period of time and parents barely have a chance to grieve for one child before they are confronted with the reality of sickness with another one. These feelings can be overwhelming when parents lack the support system needed to help them manage the parenting routine as family dynamics begin to change.

While the following stories may share emotions and experiences that can be difficult to think about, most of the mothers I've worked with in writing this book express an overall feeling of strength that is born from managing the challenges they face on a daily basis. I believe that these women have the power to remind us that it's ok to be weak from time to time. Not a single one claims to be Superwoman, but they all most certainly are outstanding mothers.

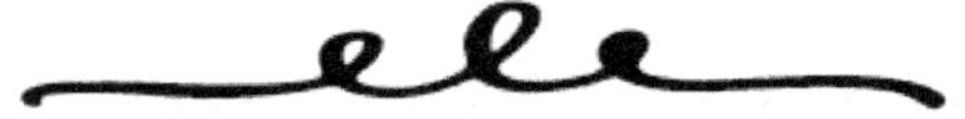

The Murphy Family: Unique Challenges of Military Life

The fact that Myra is a military wife, often called on to care for her boys as a single-parent while her husband Jordan is away on deployment, is reason enough for honoring her with Supermom status. But in the year following her youngest son Weston's diagnosis, she would be faced with many more challenges than the average soldier's wife would have to know.

With what they thought was the worst behind them, the Murphys danced into 2012 feeling pretty good. Baby Weston was recovering nicely from his bout with DKA and Myra and Jordan were starting to feel more at ease with their roles caring for a Type 1 toddler. As a result, the holidays seemed to be filled with extra cheer. Myra sported a cute sassy hairdo ready for a bright new year. The uncharacteristically warm Chicago winter meant extra fresh air and outdoor exercise for Myra and her three boys, yielding a reprieve from the cabin fever they usually suffered at this time of year. Things were looking up.

But the good feelings would only last so long. 2012 would soon prove to be a long year of struggles for medical supplies and return trips to the hospital for too many Murphy family members.

"I'm so upset right now," Myra recounts in a Facebook entry on January 3. "We found out today that Weston has been denied for getting the insulin pump. Not just a temporary denial, but until he is 7! I'm so sorry my husband has served in the military for almost the last 20 years so that when we need medical care for our child it can be denied. Yesterday we were told Weston wasn't active for prescription stuff anymore either. WTF!!"

While experiences vary, too often, military families struggle to get medical supplies that people on private insurance have an easier time acquiring. As with many other things in the world of disease management, experiences are often based on luck. The Murphy family's push to get Weston on a pump so soon after diagnosis is not the popular course of action for parents of young diabetic children (but having to wait four years to be eligible is also quite extreme).

According to a 2014 study, insulin pump use by children over the age of 6 is higher in the US than in other countries, averaging about 47% [which is still less than half] as opposed to roughly 40% in Austria and Germany and roughly 15% in England and Wales (Maahs). While I haven't been able to find an exact number for infants and toddlers, it's reasonable to assume that the percentage of younger diabetics on pumps is much lower since England's pump statistics drop to less than half for the pre-school age group, coming in at around 6%.

There are many reasons for this. Some doctors actively discourage pump use in the early months urging parents to get comfortable managing the basics first. As my husband and I were strongly warned in the hospital, "What happens if you find yourself on vacation and the pump fails and you can't get backup supplies? In most parts of the world you can get needles and insulin, but they're not much good to you if you don't know how to use them." We heeded that warning and didn't even bring the topic of conversation up again for many months.

Other times parents are hesitant to attach objects to their baby's body. Sometimes this is because they simply don't want to draw attention to their child's medical condition; other times it's due to simple lack of real estate. My son's pod (part of the Omnipod system which uses "pods" to store insulin directly on the body) is 1 ½ inches wide. His arm is 2 ½ inches wide (at best when squished). The surface of the pod is a flat piece of plastic which doesn't always work well with little curved body parts. From an engineering perspective, the system just doesn't work. As a result, we wind up attaching pods to his belly (a site which we are repeatedly reminded is "not FDA approved"). He's pretty lean, so there's not much space there either, but the belly seems to suffer fewer of the bangs and bumps that dislodge pods from arm and leg sites, so we go with it.

Some parents, like the Murphys, go with a wired pump such as the Medtronic, which has a smaller surface at the attachment site. This type of unit poses it's own set of problems as tubes can get kinked or disconnected. And because little ones have to carry the pump around with them in a fanny pack (or SPIbelt® like what many runners use) all day, there are instances where they manage to do damage to the pump or change the settings—modern designs and parent ingenuity minimize this risk, but it still exists.

And of course, another reason some parents forgo the pump is cost. Some parents can't get approval from insurance at all, in which case the expense of the pump is usually prohibitive. Prices as of 2016 were roughly $1200 to get started on the Omnipod system and $400 monthly maintenance or $5,000-$6,000 to get started with other systems, but with monthly maintenance costs under $100. Like most other things medically related, prices will likely change, but in the roughly 40 years that this type of equipment has been available, it has always fit into the category of "expensive".

Even with insurance, the cost can be too much for families on a tight budget. When we first got started with the Omnipod System (with assistance from our insurance) we laid out about $400 (in 2014) to get started and $80 per month for a monthly shipment of replacement pods. That price stayed consistent for the two years that he was on the system. For us it was a struggle but one we could manage. For some families, it's just not an option.

Eventually, with a little persistence from Myra and an agreement to hold off on the continuous glucose monitoring system, Weston was able to get his pump, with insurance covering a good deal of the costs.

"This is my new MPP player," he proudly told everyone, recognizing that his pump sack was just like his big brothers' MP3 player pouches.

January passed rather quickly, with Myra and her husband Jordan attending regular training sessions with the diabetic educator. It was their understanding that Jordan would be leaving for his deployment in the spring, and they wanted to be sure that Myra was fully prepared to manage Weston's care on her own. But as the month came to an end, so did the promise of a bright new year. Jordan had to spend two weeks away from the family (part of his Reserves duty), leaving Myra to manage the boys on her own. With Weston starting to potty-train, two school-age boys to help with homework, and stress of round-the-clock finger checks without her husband's help, there was enough for Myra to worry about without added complications.

"At one point I had to figure out how to help Weston potty train with a pump pouch permanently wrapped around his waist," Myra recalls. Helping a little guy shoot and aim without an obstructed view is hard enough—throwing a piece of medical baggage in Weston's line of sight threw an added challenge into the exercise.

But as the Chicago winter started to show its true potential and the snow barreled down on the city of Plainfield, these trivial obstacles would start to seem insignificant. At the end of February, Weston's older brother Daxton was brought to the urgent care center with yet another bout of strep throat (he had suffered at least four in recent months, along with several double ear infections). Fortunately for Myra, she had to stay home with Daxton's brothers, leaving Jordan to manage the visit without her. When they got to the center, Jordan and Daxton met up with the same doctor that had diagnosed Weston with diabetes just two months earlier.

"I refer to the experience as a significant emotional event," Jordan says. "I had a hard time maintaining my composure." Many parents have a tough time driving by the hospital where their child was treated; Jordan was forced to relive the moment firsthand, walking past the room where he had learned that his son's life would never be the same.

And this was only the beginning of the struggles. On March 16th, Weston's older brother, ten-year-old Hayden, bravely marched into the Quest lab, wearing his Fighting Irish t-shirt as he prepared for his blood to be drawn and sent to Trialnet—a medical screening facility out of the University of Florida, which screens siblings and immediate relatives of Type 1 diabetics for their likelihood of developing the disease. Within two weeks, the Murphys would learn that he had tested positive for three out of four autoantibodies for Type 1 diabetes, and that "it was not a matter of if he would get the disease, but when." As of the writing of this book (several years after my initial interview with Myra), Hayden is still diabetes-free. While nobody can predict the future, this does worth mentioning as it can provide hope to those who might be sitting around "waiting for the other shoe to drop."

While many parents wait nervously for those results to come back, the Murphys barely had time to think about it. Within that brief window of time, while still nursing Daxton back to health from his battle with strep, Myra was informed that Hayden had "walking pneumonia" and she would be without Jordan's help again for a while because his appendix needed to come out--immediately! The one highlight to this experience was that it meant a delay before his deployment.

Three days after the surgery, Myra was left caring for baby Weston who was sick with a fever—always a concern for diabetics as it makes it so much more difficult to keep blood sugars in a safe range.

"I hope someone deals Myra a good hand soon," her loving husband Jordan pleaded on his Facebook page. "On top of dealing with my surgery and recovery, she had to take Weston to the doctor this morning because he is running a fever and wheezing. She is the best ever, and deserves a friggin' break." As desperately as he wanted to help her, there was nothing he could do, confined to bed rest, still recovering from his recent appendectomy.

Less than a week later Myra was back in the emergency room with Hayden who was having trouble breathing, and back again a few days later to follow up with Jordan's surgeon.

"You know you've had too many family members in the hospital lately when you remember what is good on the hospital menu," Myra declared. Indeed. And they still hadn't even gotten the bad news back from Hayden's Trialnet screening.

Eventually, the combination of stress and fatigue would be too much for Myra, landing her on mandated bed rest along with her boys. Sometimes even moms have to give in for a while.

After a few days of bed rest, Myra was feeling physically better but still emotionally drained as she tried to pull herself together to prepare for the Easter holiday. As she walked the aisles of Target, looking for Easter basket treats that wouldn't make managing Weston's diabetes an added nightmare, she finally lost control and gave in to a complete emotional breakdown.

"I want him to feel normal… It just makes me so sad that all these damn holidays are about candy!" she exclaimed to her Facebook friends as she recalled the event. In the weeks that followed, as she was able to find a little emotional distance from the moment joked, "I probably looked like I was an abused woman walking behind Jordan, sobbing."

Soon enough, Easter and the long spring break that had everyone home, would come and go. The boys each had new Cubs jerseys from their Easter baskets to wear as they prepared for baseball season, and it was back to life as usual as the two older boys returned to school. Spring was in the air, and with temperatures in the high seventies and even eighties throughout much of March, tulips were in full bloom state-wide. It seemed things might be turning around for the Murphys.

Unfortunately, once again, they found the carefree life to be short-lived. Within a few days of returning to school, Daxton presented with a severe allergic reaction to his strep throat antibiotics and had to be switched to the stronger Prednisone. A week later, with still no recovery in sight, it was determined that he would need to have his tonsils and adenoids removed and tubes put in his ears (to prevent the recurring ear infections he had been suffering through between bouts of strep).

By this time, the calm warm weather that had characterized early spring in Chicagoland was evolving into one of the most catastrophic tornado seasons in history—a trend which seemed to mirror the upheaval in the Murphy home. Fortunately, the distractions of Father's Day and closely spaced birthdays for Daxton and Weston helped lift spirits in the month of June.

With the heat of July and August came plenty of opportunities for the distractions of summer—backflips in the pool for the older boys, and a loss of water wings for little Weston; trips to the aquarium, zoo, Museum of Science and Industry, and even a day trip to Lincoln's home and tomb in Springfield.

Compared to a very trying spring and busy summer, the fall months seemed uneventful for most of the family members. Unfortunately, Myra's mom's dog Pepper, a beautiful chocolate lab, was diagnosed with a severe case of pancreatitis—a strange coincidence considering the diabetic shadow hanging over the household. After a series of attempted medical treatments, and an extended stay at the vet, she lost her battle and died in surgery. It was an emotionally difficult time for the family, and as they approached Weston's "diaversary"—a term coined by diabetic families to mark the anniversary of the date of diagnosis—a general sense of melancholy and reflection set in as Myra looked to the turn of another year.

At some moments Myra and Jordan would find themselves overwhelmed by the anger and despair that inevitably strikes parents of young diabetic children. "This is what our lives revolve around," Jordan unloaded on his Facebook page one November day. "Stabbing a 3-year-old in the hand 8-10 times a day. Hoping and praying that the number that shows up on the screen will be in range. Waking up at 2 am every day just to make sure his blood sugar isn't low enough to kill him in his sleep. Hoping he doesn't have a bad site so that his blood sugar doesn't skyrocket. No one controls Type 1 diabetes, it controls you. You do what IT says, when it says it. Neither my wife nor my son has had a break from this for 11 months. He has been stabbed in the hand no less than 2600 times in the last 11 months... Type 1 makes you re-evaluate everything... Type 1 makes you glad as F*UCK you are married to Myra Mackie Murphy, who does this every day, no matter what, because she knows what can happen if it isn't dealt with properly."

Jordan's angry tone echoes the feelings of every parent of a diabetic child at one point or another. The online support pages cry out with such rantings. Only to be answered with the heartfelt condolences of other parents who know the feelings too well: "Hang in there, I know where you're coming from"..."We have days like that too, tomorrow will be better"...Let it out, we're here for you."

And the words of encouragement are true—diabetes can bring days of empowerment that might not otherwise be known in a life without struggle. "Type 1 diabetes is a gift," Myra stated later that month—almost in defiance of the emotions that were strangling the couple a few weeks earlier. "It has truly made me realize what is important in life. It has shown me that my three besties are the best friends anyone could ask for. Whether it is listening to me cry, offering me encouragement or getting in the trenches with me, these ladies have done it. And it has made my marriage to Jordan stronger. I would not be where I am today in my diabetes management if I hadn't had him there with me the first week home from the hospital, when he mastered shots & finger pokes and all I could do every time I looked at Weston was run into the other room to cry. It has given me wonderful new friends that I wouldn't have met any other way."

Myra's positive outlook at the end of that year is cause enough for celebration. Living life with "an invisible disease", as most people have come to regard diabetes, is difficult in that people on the outside of the close circle of family and friends tend to dismiss the severity of the condition. "At least its not cancer" is one of the well-intentioned, but heartless condolences that many of us have come to hear too many times. "If you only knew..." is what most of us would love to reply back, if only we weren't so overcome with exhaustion and frustration in such moments. In instances where close family and friends are equally dismissive, the pain upon hearing such brush-offs is even more searing.

Myra and Jordan are fortunate in that they have a strong family unit, with help from parents and close friends. They are lucky that they have grown stronger and more loving in their relationship since their son was diagnosed with Diabetes, whereas many families are torn apart by the disease. A number of different studies have found the divorce rate to be about 20-30% higher than the national 50% average for couples caring for a child with special needs. In other words, roughly 70-80% of relationships that involve such high-level care will end in divorce.

Add to this the fact that Jordan is in the military and the family constantly lives under the shadow of preparing for deployment, and the pair seem more like something out of a fairytale romance than the couple down the block. But they're doing it. They're supporting each other and loving each other, and figuring out a way to raise their boys in the most positive environment possible. True to their vows, they are in this thing called life "for better or for worse, and in sickness and in health." As Myra so aptly pointed out, now they can fairly wait for the richer parts of life they were promised to live through together.

Unfortunately, as Myra might eventually learn, should her son Hayden develop Type 1, having a second child diagnosed with the disease changes the family dynamic in a whole new way. Heather, mother of Seth and Sayde knows this all too well.

As she explained to me regretfully when we spoke, "My kids never really learned to swim because the [insulin] pump pieces would always fall off in the water, so eventually, we just stopped taking them to the pool." It's just one of the many heartbreaks she shares of life with diabetes.

~ Happy Updates ~

In reviewing this story for publication (8 years after her initial interview), Myra pointed out that Hayden actually qualified for a TrialNet clinical trial as a result of his screening results. During the trial, he was given a course of oral insulin, but the study was discontinued early and determined to be a failed trial. Fortunately, as of this writing, Hayden is still diabetes-free. Also, the following year, as I prepared to relaunch this book under a new title, Myra reached out to let me Westin and his siblings most definitely did learn how to swim. I've decided to keep the initial interview quote in the story because it speaks to how desperate things can feel in the early days, just following diagnosis. But it also goes to show how much can change over the years. Hopefully, this update serves as a strong glimmer of hope to those who are still learning to navigate "their new normal" in relation to diabetes.

Heather, Sayde & Seth: Managing the Care of Two Young Diabetics

At some point in the journey, all Type 1 parents will come to identify certain ways in which normalcy is traded out in favor of "the numbers". Even when we all echo the mantra of "kid first, diabetes second," there come times when we opt for easier glucose control over the free-and-easy lifestyle. Living in Hawaii, my family and I spend a lot of time at the beach and the pool. Which means Connor spends a good deal of time around water. When he was little, and just learning to swim, we would keep his dex (his continuous monitor) on his arm to minimize the amount of time it would be fully submersed in water. We would also plan beach days around his "pod" (insulin-pump)-change days so that we rarely went to the beach with a new pod on his body. He hasn't been on a pump for a few years now, but we used to change the pods out every three days--so two out of every three days were generally non-water activity days. I rarely, if ever, brought him to the beach immediately following a site change, because I knew that the new piece would likely fall off (or become filled with sand and have to be pulled off), making it a complete waste.

Fortunately, I only have one child to manage this way, and the sacrifice isn't too burdensome. I can't even imagine how much more difficult this juggling act would become if I had two children (with two separate sets of equipment) to manage.

"People say it gets easier but even after all this time, all I can think when I hear those words is how can you say that?" Heather told me. It's been nearly eight years since I interviewed her, but there are some things that seem to be eternal truths in a Type 1 parent's world. At the time, she said she still couldn't bring herself to tell people that it gets easier "because I can't bring myself to lie to them. Sure, some things get easier, but then other things just get harder."

Listening to Heather share her experiences, then eight years after her youngest daughter Sayde was diagnosed with Type 1, was incredibly moving. Even after all the years that have passed since we last spoke, I can still remember her beautiful Southern drawl--the way it made me feel like I could pull up a rocker, pour some lemonade, and listen to her for hours. "I've thought about writing our story but it's just too hard," she told me. "Every time I try, I just get too emotional."

Sayde, then ten, had been diagnosed with Type 1 when she was only 18 months old. As Heather explained to me, she and her family are Cherokee and while Type 2 Diabetes is quite common in the Cherokee community, Type 1 is not. And so, as with many parents, Type 1 Diabetes just wasn't a concern that was on Heather's radar. Unfamiliar with the warning signs in young children and unsuspecting of the disease in her own daughter, by the time Heather and her husband got Sayde to the hospital, her blood sugar was in the 800s, and she was in DKA. Because Sayde's condition was so tenuous, she needed to be medevacked to a children's hospital in another state.

After reviewing this story for publication, Heather messaged me, "I want to add something about how when Sayde was flown to Arkansas Children's Hospital, it was on a donated plane from a private individual . I wish I could find and thank them." The reality is that most families don't have supplemental insurance riders to cover things like medivac flights. Even a basic ambulance ride can set families back thousands of dollars. I can't help but pause to think about the strong surge of emotions that must have been coursing through Heather at the moment she learned a complete stranger was going to pay for the life-saving flight her daughter needed.

Fortunately, when Sayde's older brother Seth was diagnosed six months later, Heather and her husband Jayme had gained enough knowledge to avoid the same traumatic experience they had suffered through with Sayde. Seth was nearing his fourth birthday when they started to notice the all-too-familiar symptoms of excessive thirst and bathroom runs. When they took Seth to the hospital, his blood sugar was only 180 and he was not in DKA. Heather choked up as she explained that while Seth's diagnosis should have been easier, emotionally, it was actually much harder.

There was no emergency flight to the children's hospital, and three-year-old Seth, who was in relatively good health at the time of diagnosis—other than early symptoms of diabetes—was able to pass his time in the newly remodeled endocrinology ward playing video games for hours on end. But as they packed up the car for the three-hour drive back home, Seth asked the one question that broke his mother's heart: "Does this mean that I'm like Sayde now?"

Heather cried just recounting the moment and explained, "He didn't say it with any resentment in his voice, but it was obvious that he knew what it meant to have diabetes, and that he grasped how much his life was about to change. He knew about having to measure every meal before it was eaten and about having to get injections every day. I just cried."

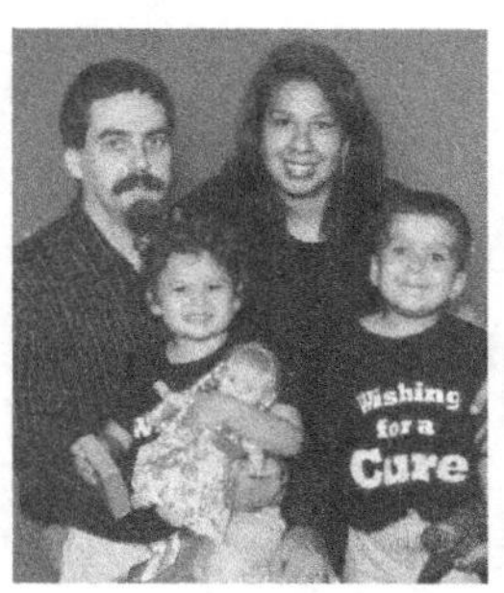

The early days following Sayde and Seth's diagnosis, at a JDRF gala event in Tulsa, OK

Even when Sayde was first diagnosed, Heather had an inkling of what life with diabetes would be like. In grade school, she was good friends with a girl Paige, who had also been diagnosed with Type 1 at the same age as Sayde--18 months old. By the time she and Heather had become friends, Paige was fairly capable of managing her diabetes independently, counting her carbs at lunchtime and adjusting insulin based on food intake and activity level. "She was super competitive and we rivaled each other in everything," Heather told me. "But I always knew when to back off. Everyone always knew when she wasn't feeling well, and then there was nothing we could really do. She would just get super moody until she was feeling better."

Recalling the years with Paige, and specifically, her resistance to talking about the disease around friends, reminded Heather of the differences between her own two kids. Heather explained that while Sayde had always seemed comfortable showing off her pump supplies and equipment—happy to do her part to educate the public about the realities and misconceptions of Type 1 Diabetes—Seth was quite the opposite. Like Paige, Seth would shut down when asked about his diabetes. He didn't want to talk about it, and he covered up any part of his body where a pump or glucose monitor might have been seen.

When the kids were first offered the opportunity to go on the Dex (when Seth was eleven), he resisted. "That was his choice," Heather explained. "I wasn't going to force either of them to wear another piece of equipment if they didn't want to." Sayde was the first to start using the Dex. She actually wanted it. Seth held back for a good month before offering to give it a try. "But my a1c better be a lot better by my next appointment," Seth demanded, "or I'm taking it off!"

Hearing this story from Heather so many years ago (when Connor was still a toddler), I couldn't really comprehend the meaning of all that she was telling me. But now, having a spirited 10-year-old diabetic of my own, I get it. Connor is allowed to make choices about his equipment, just as Heather has allowed Seth and Sayde to make such medical decisions themselves. It's the reason Connor is "MDI" (or on Multiple Daily Injections) instead of on a pump. Because, as we've both come to realize, we parents are only temporary caretakers. Ultimately, the responsibility for disease management will rest with the individual themselves. Empowering them to make important decisions early on enables them to make critical decisions down the road.

On a basic level, it might seem like a blessing to have a spunky child-like Seth, who demanded results from such burdensome medical equipment. Why should anyone pay (financially, physically, or otherwise) for equipment that fails to deliver on its promises? But such strong-will in a diabetic child can be challenging as well. Heather knew that the benefits of continuous glucose monitoring would extend well beyond respectable a1c levels and that it could take years to realize the real benefits of such technology. But as she explained, she also "never wanted to scare the kids about things like organ failure or blindness that [could] result from poorly managed diabetes." But at the same time, she wondered how she could "get him to realize that tools like the Dex can literally save his life and protect his body from long-term damage if I don't talk to him about serious diabetes-related complications?"

Heather was right. The control that comes from using a continuous monitor simply can not be duplicated with intermittent finger sticks—at least not for children. Some adults are able to keep their blood sugar fairly steady by sticking to regular doses of insulin and keeping a regimented diet with little variation from day to day. That type of lifestyle is incredibly difficult with young children, and even when managed, variables like growth spurts and common colds make regular fine-tuning of insulin calculations a must.

Such frequent adjustments (facilitated by continuous glucose monitoring) can be a nuisance, but the benefits pay off, both in the short-term with lowered a1c levels, and later down the road. But many of the benefits are unseen by young kids like Seth, with the payoff coming not in months, but in years. It takes time for the diabetic child to see any rewards for daily sacrifices, and Seth will likely be in his thirties or forties by the time he can appreciate finding himself with a lower-than-average risk for heart disease or kidney failure than the average diabetic.

"And what I really wish he would understand," Heather pointed out to me, "is that access to this technology isn't a burden—it's a privilege. I know a mom who is paying $1200 per month for a Dex for her daughter because insurance won't cover the supplies. The girl is going through puberty and with wildly fluctuating hormones, they're having a tough time controlling her blood sugar." With a small hint at humor, Heather added, "I told Seth, 'I love you, but there's no way I would pay $1200 a month for you to be on a Dex. You don't know how lucky you are!"

But how does a mother truly get across such concepts to a pre-teen? Heather shared a conversation that she had had with the kids' orthodontist. Seth had asked the doctor if he had to get braces. To which the doctor responded, "Son, you don't have to have anything. You can wait until you're older and can pay for it yourself." Seth, like most kids at that age, wasn't able to grasp the full impact of immediate choices on long-term outcomes. Whether it's braces, glasses, or insulin supplies, providing such tools on an ongoing basis is often a financial and logistical nightmare for parents (some traveling hours each way to secure such supplies), but they willingly make the sacrifice because they know that it's what's best for their child. In the case of braces, if adolescent Seth had failed to visualize life as a twenty-something-year-old with crooked teeth, and decided to forgo the braces, the worst that would happen would be that he would be left kicking himself for his stupidity down the road, with the upside being that he would have saved his mom quite a bit of hassle and money throughout his high school years. Should he have failed to take advantage of the offer of the Dexcom however, the long-term implications could potentially be much more severe.

Managing diabetes in an older child certainly presents challenges quite different from caring for an infant or toddler. Most parents who are inducted into the world of Type-1 parenting when their child is young find themselves torn between eagerly awaiting the days when the child is old enough to understand the implications of sneaking food, and dreading the time that will surely come when the maturing child starts demanding independence and freedom to make choices. As Heather pointed out, "Some things get easier, but then other things just get harder."

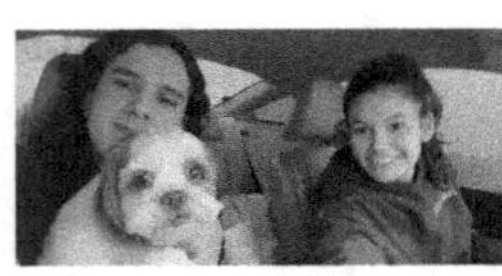

This image is a testament to how hard Heather has worked over the years to keep two Type 1 children healthy and strong

Heather reflected on some earlier days—before adolescent hormones and streaks of independence complicated diabetes management. Even when the kids were less self-aware and the reality of being different from other kids held less weight, just going every-day places with two diabetic children posed challenges that most parents could never understand. There always had to be enough insulin on hand to account for highs in both kids, and enough sugar to account for double lows. And of course, things could break (pumps fail and insulin bottles break), and juices can spill. As Heather said, "You have to have a backup for the backup."

She told me about a time they drove twelve hours to see the air show in Pensacola. "After a short time in the heat, both kids were dropping dangerously low and I didn't have enough sugar to treat both of them." After cutting the concession line to get Gatorade for the kids and taking the time to bring both of their levels back into safe ranges, (both of their blood sugars had been in the 20s!), she found that they had missed almost the entire show. Even though Heather had had the help of her husband and the kids' grandparents while she ran around trying to gather extra supplies, in the end, the only way to put an end to the stress of the day was to just go home. She convinced some event workers to drive her and the kids to the main gate, hoping to avoid any additional crashes, and they all called it a day.

It's experiences like this that have more experienced Type 1 parents explaining to those who are newer to this reality, that if you ever take your kids to a place like Disney, don't feel an ounce of guilt in asking for the disability pass. When you have to take your child out of a line that you've been standing in for over an hour (because there's no other way to treat the low), you'll be grateful to have it!

Heather also shared an experience that took place at an amusement park a little closer to home. She remembered how even when over-packing (as she thought they had) with extra pump supplies, insulin, backup syringes, and simple carbs, it's still possible to come up short. "I brought five boxes of supplies and went through all of them," Heather explained. "One kid's pump failed with a No Delivery alarm, and the disposable applicators kept falling off. When we ran out of pump supplies, we switched to shots, but we eventually ran out of those too. Then we just had to go home."

Throughout our entire time chatting, as she sifted through all of the bittersweet memories, her attitude was always positive--even when sharing the regretful experiences that would send most parents into a complete tizzy. "One time, I even gave the wrong kid a shot," she told me. Obviously, that's not a worry for most parents. But even recounting such stressful moments, Heather always focused on the positives--especially in regard to the hope to be found in modern diabetes research.

For example, Heather's friend Lauren, who she met through the local JDRF chapter, was one of the first individuals to be fitted with an artificial pancreas. This technology was still in early trial phases at the time, and as of December 2015, Lauren was just one of ten individuals in the world to have one.

According to a 2015 edition of Diabetes Forecast, "the artificial pancreas bridges the gap between two pieces of diabetes technology that already exist: the insulin pump and the continuous glucose monitor..."

Because it's been nearly eight years now since I first wrote this review (because such is the life of a Type 1 parent), a lot has changed in the world of diabetes management. As it turns out, I never cited this article properly the first time around, and now can't find it because Diabetes Forecast doesn't even exist as a publication anymore. But these changes also help highlight what Heather was emphasizing at the time--there is so much research being done in relation to diabetes care, that it can be difficult (in a good way) to keep up with all the changes. The difference between what was available in 1920 vs. 2020 is similar to the advances made in space travel during that same time. While the artificial pancreas (or anything similar) seemed like an unreachable dream for the average person back in 2015, now, in 2022 there are multiple "closed loop" systems that allow for communication between a person's continuous glucose monitor (cgm) and their pump. Connor is even considering going back to pumping just to try it!

This technology is still far from a cure—only when a person no longer has the disease can it be said that they are cured--and it is not even that revolutionary. Insulin pumps have been around and evolving for roughly sixty years and continuous glucose monitors are now entering their third decade. But by marrying the two technologies together (and making that technology increasingly available to the general public), developers have found a way to reduce the risk of human error and improve on the functionality of both devices.

The "closed loop" systems that are becoming more readily available are different from the "artificial pancreas," which at last search included a second pump to distribute glucagon when blood sugars are low. Because the technologies are developing faster than a Type 1 mom can effectively research and write a book, the best way to stay on top of the most recent advances is to attend conferences and/or follow the research online as it comes out [4].

Again, as exciting as the new technologies are, they are still far from perfect--pumps still fall off at the beach, cannulas get clogged, and everyday sibling rough-housing still results in ripped-off CGMs. But for patients like Lauren (Heather's good friend from the JDRF conference), closed-loop systems are a dramatic step in the right direction. According to Lauren, in her interview with NWA News back in 2015, in the first few months of being fitted with the artificial pancreas, her blood sugar levels remained steady day and night, regardless of what she ate or how active she was (the two factors which make stabilizing blood sugar a regular challenge). She said she felt like she could finally appreciate what it might be like to live a life without diabetes.

Fortunately, JDRF is actively engaged in raising funds for research and technological development, and the race for a cure has never been stronger. In that regard, it is likely that by the time most people have access to technology like this, it will already be obsolete, with newer and more advanced devices being worked on. For people like Heather, even if her children never see technology like the artificial pancreas, just knowing that so much energy is being poured into improving the lives of Type 1 diabetics is a reason for hope.

In addition to finding hope in the research and technological advancements for diabetes management, Heather also thought it was important to emphasize that her strong faith in God is what has kept her sane over the years. While I have made a conscious effort to minimize the number of religious references within each of the stories so that they can serve as a source of inspiration for the broadest audience possible, I do also believe it's important to honor the voices of each individual as accurately as possible. But as Heather so accurately points out, "Diabetes doesn't care about your bank account, skin color, [religion] or education!!!"; as such, each parent needs to find their strength in any and all spaces available.

Footnotes: 1. Heather's friend's name was changed to protect her privacy. 2. An a1c is a blood test that gives doctors an idea of how well blood sugars have been managed over a 3-month period of time. This will be defined in the glossary, so a specific note here will likely not be needed. 3. Lauren Sivewright's name remains unchanged as her story has been publicly broadcast on NWA news out of Fayetteville, AR. 4. The most current pediatric CGMs on the market at the time of the original writing were the Minimed by Medtronic or the G5 version of the Dexcom. Many patients were still using older versions of these CGMs due to insurance setbacks or uncertainty about certain issues with the newest versions. 5. 6. There are a number of insulin pumps on the market, but the ones most commonly discussed on the pediatric diabetes support groups at the time were the Animas Ping and Omnipod. Parents seemed to like the Animas because they could "bolus" or direct the pump to deliver insulin from up to 10 feet away (convenient for working with toddlers on the run), it was waterproof up to 12 feet, and because the insulin was stored in a unit which was not directly attached to the body, the applicator which attached to the skin was relatively small and easy to fit on the smaller body parts of children. One of the drawbacks to this pump was that the computer that directs insulin delivery was attached to the body with a tube and had to be carried close to the body at all times (usually with the help of a "fanny-pack") so parents worried about tubes kinking or being torn off by active toddlers. Omnipod users (then and now) like the "pods" for their lack of tubing and the fact that they are waterproof to 26 feet. Some drawbacks to this system are that the pods must be changed every 2-3 days and they are larger than site attachments on wired pumps (because they must store the insulin), which can make them difficult to attach to small infant/toddler body parts.

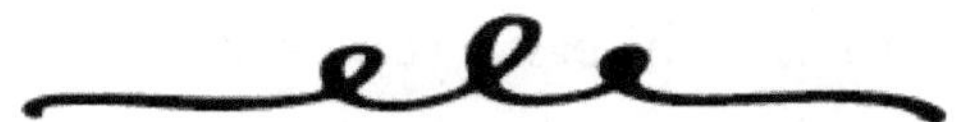

Jessica & Oliver: Managing Diabetes with an Insulin Allergy

Jessica originally shared her story with me in 2016, just as I was finishing up my master's program in creative writing and looking forward to a possible PhD program in adolescent literacy. In my heart, I knew that the stories of the moms I had spoken with needed to be shared, but there was a big part of me that needed to reclaim myself a bit as well. At that point, we had been living with diabetes for roughly 2 1/2 years. Connor had a full-time nurse at school, and I was starting to see myself as having an identity beyond care-giver again. I had long toyed with the idea of getting my PhD, but I was finally starting to feel adventurous enough to do so. Unfortunately, that meant that many of the stories I had been working on got pushed to the side as I started to first study for the GRE, then muddle my way through the whole application process, and eventually go on to tackle new studies.

Eventually, in January of 2017, I moved with my family from Maui to Columbia, South Carolina, where I would embark on my new journey. I started to tackle the book project again on the side and was excited to be diving back into the stories each woman had so graciously shared with me. Unfortunately, the move didn't work out for our family, and 6 months later, we moved back to Maui. There is a lot more to the story of what has happened to us in the past 8 years, but in short-form, this book project wound up at the bottom of a very deep pile of other, more pressing priorities. As a result, Jessica and Oliver's story sat neglected in a dusty corner of my "BF and Diabetes Book Project" file for far too long.

It is now 2022. I recently reached out to Jessica to see if she would still be interested in having her story featured in the book. She responded with enthusiasm: "Yes, Absolutely!" All she asked was that I update her email address because she had divorced in the years since we had last touched base. She has also launched a website with a handful of other women to raise awareness about Oliver's rare allergy to insulin and put herself through nursing school while managing Oliver's care as a single mom.

As with so many of the families that I have connected with in the T1 community over the years, Jessica and Oliver's lives had changed dramatically over the course of just a few short years. Maybe that's the way it is with all lives—nobody's life just stands still because you lose touch with them for a few years—but somehow Type-1 families seem to live a lifetime of joy, grief and growth in the brief periods that many others seem to consider just a blip on the map of time. And it is for this reason, that I've chosen to share the following portion of Jessica and Oliver's story in the chapter on Changing Family Dynamics, as opposed to keeping it with the rest of her story in the chapter on Breastfeeding at Diagnosis,

Oliver is now eight years old. He is no longer the little nursling that he was when Jessica and I first connected. Some of Oliver's journey is captured on IAHAwareness.Org, a website dedicated to educating others about insulin allergies and hypersensitivities. These conditions are rare, but when they do present, they make the challenges of managing diabetes care exponentially more complicated.

Oliver experienced his first negative reaction to synthetic insulin when he was three years old—roughly 18 months after his initial diagnosis. Unfortunately, this condition is so rare, that many doctors were stumped by what was going on. After countless doctor's appointments and lab visits, Jessica finally got Oliver in to see an allergist—only to be told that insulin allergies don't exist and that she was imagining what she was seeing. As an interesting aside, PubMed.Gov (the National Library of Medicine) published a research article on this very topic in 2008 (10 years before Jessica first walked into that allergist's office). As many T1 parents have come to realize, just because the research exists, doesn't mean your doctor has read it. With so much information out there to digest, there is no way for doctors to keep up with it all. When in doubt—and whenever possible—parents should never be ashamed of doing their own research and bringing that material to doctor's appointments when they go. As it was, it would take a lot of persistence on Jessica's part, and nearly 8 months from the initial angry, red flareup on his leg, for Oliver to officially be diagnosed with an insulin allergy. And even then, the only known remedy was to put him on high doses of antihistamine to combat the flare-ups.

It has now been nearly 6 years since Jessica received confirmation of Oliver's insulin allergy, and options aren't much better. Kayla Mattingly, another board member for the IAH Awareness team was recently featured in an article in Healthline. In the article, written in 2021, Mike Hoskins explains that most allergic reactions experienced during pumping or insulin injection relate to preservatives in the insulin. The more severe and rare type of reaction is actually in response to the insulin itself and currently, there is still no effective cure or remedy. Through his article, Hoskins shares some various studies on the subject, including a 3-decade study conducted by Bzowyckyj and Stahnke (2018), but not much progress has been made. Currently, the "bandaids" that patients must resort to include things like switching to pork or beef insulins (the precursors to modern synthetic insulin) or attempting to desensitize the body through a combination of antihistamines or corticosteroids and insulin dosing. Unfortunately, animal insulins can be difficult to obtain and are not a reliable source of ongoing care, and for many patients, desensitization just doesn't seem to work. This means little kiddos like Oliver have to suffer a double dose of misery when receiving their life-giving care.

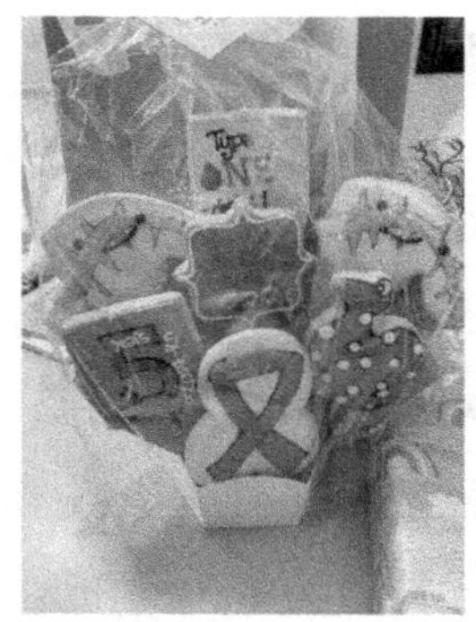

A "Diaversary Basket" with diabetes-themed cookies to celebrate the anniversary of the date Oliver was diagnosed with Type 1

What always amazes me about women like Jessica is that when life throws challenges their way, they find ways to turn those obstacles into opportunities. On December 22, 2020, just 3 days before Christmas, Jessica and Oliver not only celebrated Oliver's 5th Diaversary (replete with blue, white and neon green, diabetes-themed cookies), but they also celebrated the end of Jessica's first month in nursing school. Just one year later, they would be able to celebrate the end of Jessica's first complete year of school and as of March 2022, she is officially a registered nurse (RN).

Jessica's fortitude has obviously rubbed off on her son. Oliver is one tough kiddo. At just 5 years old, he managed his own pump site change at school, saving his mom the trouble of having to run over and do it herself. This is beyond a big deal! Connor is 10 and I still struggle to get him to give pen injections. I can't even imagine him doing a site change independently. But Jessica has obviously done an amazing job of helping Oliver build independence. As Jessica says, building independence in our Type 1 kiddos is "bittersweet". We know that building independence allows them to live life a bit more like other kids, but it's also so hard to watch them take on such a significant medical burden from a young age. Oliver is just 2 years younger than my own son Connor, and they share similar Diaversaries. While our pathways have been a bit different and the break in communication so substantial, I feel like I've been on their journey with them this whole time. I've experienced firsthand what it is to watch a toddler grow toward adolescence. I've experienced Jessica's frustrations as she struggled to figure out why calculations that worked so well one day, failed to work the next. I've been there through the illnesses and traumas that have made mothering this little boy so heart-wrenchingly painful at times because in my heart, I have. And as I ebb and flow into and out of communication with the T1D forums on Facebook, I know that this is true for all of us T1 moms. When I see a mother post in distress after countless hours of fighting highs, or lows...battling through negotiations with the other caregivers in her child's life...fighting back tears after a painful interaction with some ignorant individual at her child's school...and then read the dozens—sometimes HUNDREDS—of comments in response, I am reminded that none of us are alone in managing this disease. We are an army of warriors out there, all waiting to lift each other up in times of distress and all woefully able to say, "I've been there."

As I reread Jessica's early communications to me, I can feel her pain as if it is my own and I am reminded of just how complex the sea of emotions are in those early days around diagnosis. She starts off her email to me by retracing the desperation and grief she lived through as she tried to make sense of Oliver's increasing frailty—and how desperately she needed to convey the devastation she had been feeling in the month before his diagnosis. As much as I needed to write this book to process my own grief, Jessica needed to share her pain with someone she knew could understand. And I do. Painfully so.

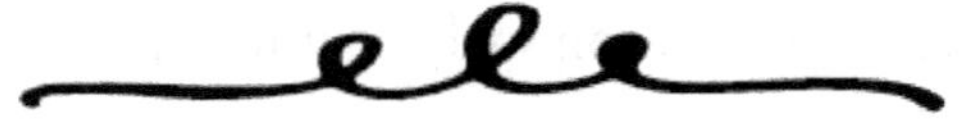

Chapter Five

Caring for the Child with Multiple Conditions

While most people would agree that managing a single life-threatening condition is sufficient in terms of building character, the unfortunate reality is that auto-immune diseases (which Type 1 diabetes is) often come in pairs—or even triplicate. Usually, there is a break between diagnoses, with the first presenting months, or even years before the arrival of subsequent conditions. Even so, the blow is rarely easy to absorb.

When we were first told that Connor had celiac and would need to go gluten-free, I would describe our mindset as mildly distressed. We didn't like the idea of managing another condition, but we shrugged our shoulders and asked, how bad can it be? Within minutes I was back in my "safe place"—the Diapers and Diabetes board—to see if others could lend some insight. One of the other moms let me know about another support group, designed for parents of kids with Type 1 and celiac together, and helped get me admitted to the group. The name of the Facebook group has changed a little over the years. Currently, it is called Empowering Parents of Children with Celiac Disease and Type 1 Diabetes. As of this current writing (December 2022), there are over 3,000 members.

When I first learned about the group, I was relieved to find out that there was another place where I'd be able to go with questions and frustrations, and took comfort in knowing that with the new diagnosis, we had the solution to Connor's wildly fluctuating blood sugars that we had been battling in the months before. But relief quickly turned to dismay when I learned how challenging it can be to keep a child with celiac away from gluten. While some families manage to keep a split kitchen, the risk of cross-contamination is high. To minimize the risk, some people keep separate cookware and appliances (such as one toaster for cooking regular bread products, and another for toasting GF products). Other families choose to convert the whole household to a GF-safe zone. This is certainly the safest option and the more practical method for the person in charge of meal preparation, but it is also much more costly than allowing non-celiac family members to continue eating normally since GF products are generally twice the cost of traditional ones. Either way, the solution rarely stays a source of comfort for long.

Unfortunately celiac is only one of the conditions that typically occur with diabetes. One of the moms in the T1/celiac group recently posted that her son was just diagnosed with a third disease—Hashimoto's Thyroiditis. In this disease, the body's immune system starts attacking the thyroid, just as it attacks the pancreas with Type 1 Diabetes. Management for the condition is slightly less burdensome (daily pills as opposed to shots, pumps, and hourly blood monitoring), but left untreated, it can lead to multiple complications including enlargement of the thyroid (known as goiter), heart failure, mental health issues, birth defects in babies of affected women, and even a life-threatening condition known as myxedema. Treatment may be "just a few pills," but the emotional burden of an added diagnosis is a weight that can't be measured.

I've found that some of the best information about complications associated with Hashimoto's and other auto-immune conditions can be found on the Mayo Clinic site. In any case, as any parent managing multiple conditions will quickly attest—each new condition results in an added layer of stress. The stories in this chapter reflect the unique challenges of caring for a family when multiple conditions are present.

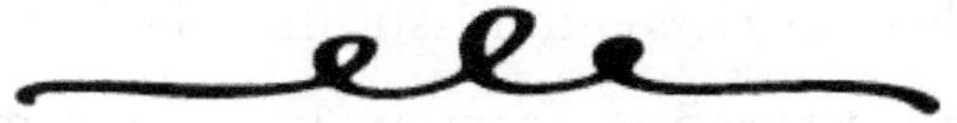

Nancy & Raymond: "I Just Can't Afford to Get Sick"

After nearly 8 years from when I first started writing this book, and roughly 5 years from when I put the last serious work into it, I decided to post a call for submissions on some of the diabetes boards again. I don't know why I was shocked, but the responses started flooding in immediately. If millions of years haven't killed the human draw to storytelling as a source of healing, it was silly of me to assume that the response to a new call for story submissions would be any less enthusiastic than the first time around.

Although this project has been a constant presence in my heart and mind over the years (especially during the months I spent interviewing women for my doctoral research on adolescent motherhood), this story--the story of Nancy and her son Raymond--represents the first freshly-written Type 1 mom story in nearly a decade.

Raymond was diagnosed in April, 2019, just six days after his first birthday. It has been 3 and 1/2 years since the diagnosis and in that time, Nancy has endured a lifetime of challenges. As I mentioned to her as we closed out her interview, it was difficult to determine the best place to fit her story because she not only has had to manage the needs of a child with multiple conditions but she has also experienced multiple "changing family dynamics" over these few short years.

Nancy's husband is a wrecker driver. I hadn't heard the term before, but as she explained to me, this means that he picks up wrecked semi-trucks and hauls them off to the body shop he works for in Rickman, TN. On the surface, this might not seem significant, but as Amanda Thames writes for The Daily News, "The average person couldn't handle the types of scenes" most wrecker drivers respond to on a regular basis. After all, wrecked vehicles (especially semis) often mean that one or more people have suffered significant injuries. Additionally, Nancy's husband spends a good percentage of his time out of town, meaning he often isn't around when challenges set in.

As Nancy prepared for our interview, she revisited old pictures and memories of when everything "went down". She shared that the mere act of looking back at those pictures was extremely emotional for her. It was a Sunday night when Raymond was diagnosed with diabetes. Nancy had her stepdaughter for the night and had planned for a small celebration with cake, but Raymond's sudden illness put those plans on hold. He was having difficulty breathing, which made Nancy initially think he was experiencing another RSV episode, like the one he had had at 9 months old.

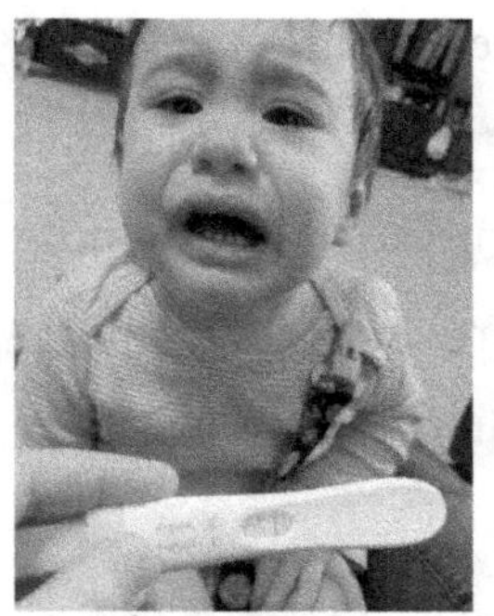

Raymond the night before his birthday, when Nancy first found out she was pregnant. Nancy describes this picture as one that gives her "massive mom guilt"

She decided to fix herself a little nest on the floor where she and Raymond could sleep together so that she could keep a close watch over him. In the morning, she fixed him a bottle but he wouldn't drink from it and he didn't even want his pacifier. "That's when I knew he was really sick," Nancy said. "I tried to carry him but he was so limp, it was like trying to carry a giant newborn." With the help of her father-in-law, Nancy was able to get Raymond and all their supplies to the hospital. There, a nurse did a blood sugar check and the result was so high that they couldn't even get a reading. However, with the use of an advanced machine, they were able to get eventually get a reading of 798. Nancy was devastated. With tears in her eyes, Nancy recalled, "I just remember bawling because I couldn't fix it."

The doctor informed her that the hospital they were at was not equipped to handle Raymond's DKA and high blood sugars, and called for an ambulance to transport them to Vanderbilt, the nearest hospital with a pediatric endocrinology ward. "I just remember looking down at Raymond in the bassinet, with his long legs hanging over the end and thinking how funny he looked," Nancy recalls. The whole experience was surreal and overwhelming for her. On the night of Raymond's diagnosis, Nancy spent her time in the ICU, hoping that her husband could make it back from Florida quickly, while she figured out how to process everything on her own. In addition to this new diagnosis, just the day before his birthday, she had taken an at-home pregnancy test and found that she was pregnant. It was a lot to make sense of with her husband so far from home.

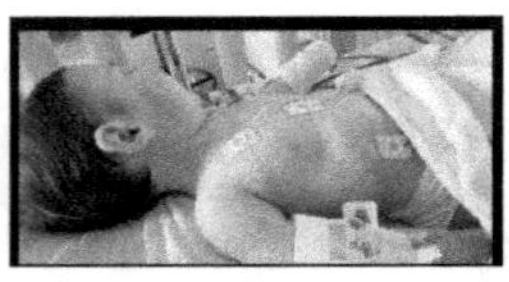

This is the only picture Nancy has from Raymond's hospital stay at the hospital. This picture was taken after Raymond was stabilized and the doctors were able to transfer the IV from his scalp to his arms.

Nancy spent those first lonely hours, struggling to find comfort in the stiff leatherette ottoman the hospital provided, for her comfort, while attempting to find some type of online resources or support. As she explains it, she was "trying to find someplace to redirect the anxiety."

And then the bleeding started. As she sat there alone, trying to process the nightmare unfolding around her one child, she also had to grieve the loss of another. To say that sometimes life can be too cruel to bear just doesn't do her experience justice. But as Nancy reminded me, sometimes just knowing that you're not alone in your struggle can be a lifeline. In those first several hours following Raymond's diagnosis, she found Scott Benner's Juicebox Podcast, and the Diapers and Diabetes group on Facebook. As Nancy remembers, "It really helped me to have somewhere to commiserate. I remember thinking, 'surely to God I'm not the only one'." As she explains, she wasn't even really looking for advice or information at that point. She just "didn't want to feel alone."

My husband and I fought like cats and dogs during our stay in the hospital with Connor. At one point, the nursing staff threatened to send one of us home if we couldn't pull ourselves together. But truth be told, I'd rather that than spending those early days alone. Even though we didn't necessarily work through the turmoil prettily, at least we worked through it together. And when one needed to take a break, they knew that the other would be keeping watch--just in case.

Nancy wasn't so fortunate. As she described to me the experience of watching the nurse insert the IV into Raymond's scalp, all I could think about was how much harder that would be to go through alone. Connor and Raymond are similar in that by the time they both arrived at the hospital, both in DKA, their veins had collapsed and traditional methods of starting an IV were not available. With Connor, they had to start the IV in his jugular. With Raymond, it was the scalp. Either scenario is quite horrific for a mother to watch. I only wish Nancy didn't have to endure that alone.

While Nancy was relieved when the opportunity finally arrived to take Raymond home, as many who have found themselves in the same situation quickly come to find out, that transition is often a rocky one. Nancy and her family live in a multi-generational home with her mother-in-law, father-in-law, sister-in-law, brother-in-law and her nephew. Her nephew is now 14 and absolutely dotes over Nancy's kids, but she recalls when she first brought Raymond home from the hospital how he asked, "What did you feed him to give him diabetes?" As Nancy shares, she knew he was just a kid and didn't mean any harm by asking the question, but "it was one of those moments when I knew, 'this is going to be hard'."

Adding to the complexity of the new family dynamic, Nancy's father-in-law is Type 2 Diabetic. While that was helpful in that it provided everyone with some familiarity with monitoring blood-sugar levels and carb intake, Type 1 and Type 2 management are extraordinarily different and those with Type 2 Diabetes may need to unlearn certain practices when learning the intricacies of caring for a child with Type 1 Diabetes. Fortunately, Nancy's father-in-law always defers to her judgment and asks for clarification if he isn't sure about something related to Raymond's care.

Unfortunately, the emotional turmoil experienced in those early days was just a hint of what was to come. In the less than 4 years since Raymond's diagnosis, he has received an additional diagnosis of celiac and is now receiving special education preschool services under the eligibility category of "Developmental Delay." As Nancy explains, Raymond was late to begin crawling and walking and is still non-verbal (at 4 1/2 years old). He was born premature, had suffered RSV prior to diagnosis, and then, at only one-year-old, suffered a significant bout of DKA. As Nancy says, "The poor guy. He just spent so long trying to get his body to do what it was supposed to do."

Fortunately, Raymond is making great progress in his new preschool program, but managing all of his needs can be emotionally exhausting. "My oldest child is 17 and neurotypical", Nancy explained to me. "RayRay is the 1st child to have all this extra stuff...and it stresses me out a little bit." She also blames herself for some of "RayRay's" lack of independence. She told me that "some of his delays are my fault because I was having a little bit of a control thing." But the "control thing" that she's talking about is so typical for parents of diabetic toddlers—especially those with insulin pumps and/or continuous monitors attached to their little bodies. It's one thing to encourage independence with a toddler when the biggest concern is getting a little pee or poop on the floor, but when devices are attached around the buttocks or abdomen (as they typically are with little ones), it can be especially stressful to watch them struggle with pants and undergarments that are likely to rip those devices off!

And as Nancy soon discovered, managing the toddler development stage would become even more challenging when pregnant and then eventually when caring for a newborn. After experiencing the heart-wrenching miscarriage in the hospital during Raymond's diagnosis, Nancy was thrilled when she discovered she was pregnant again just a few weeks after returning home. And while she considered Raymond's little sister a blessing, having a second toddler to care for while managing the complex medical needs of another can be quite overwhelming.

When it came time for Nancy to give birth, she and her husband faced the challenge that many second-time parents face in that moment--what to do with the toddler at home. In many situations, parents simply arrange for a family member or neighbor to provide care while the birthing couple is in the hospital. And in this situation, living in a multi-family home made some of those logistical challenges a bit simpler. But they still had to arrange for nighttime diabetes care which complicated matters.

When Nancy left for the hospital, her sister-in-law made a "cheat sheet" to cover the aspects of care that she wasn't comfortable with. Her sister-in-law had been helping Nancy with diabetes management for the months leading up to Ruby's birth and was comfortable with the basics, but she knew that nighttime care could present different challenges. At one point, shortly after the birth of their daughter, Nancy's husband had to leave the hospital so that he could go home and check on Raymond and help put him to bed. Ruby's birth marks the only night that Nancy has been away from Raymond since his diagnosis. Fortunately, Nancy was cleared for discharge the next day and the family returned home just in time for dinner the next evening. Raymond and his little sister Ruby are only 22 months apart. The pregnancy and early months following Ruby's birth were extremely difficult, but as Nancy points out, "Sometimes you don't have a choice but to manage." Nancy adds that she had gained a lot of weight with her second pregnancy, which made keeping up with a medically-complex toddler especially challenging.

Caring for multiple young children, especially when faced with the added challenge of medical management, can be a daunting and overwhelming task for any parent, especially for a solo-parent like Nancy. With her husband often on the road and limited support from friends who mostly work, she sometimes feels isolated in her role as a caregiver. In addition to the physical and emotional demands of being a full-time stay-at-home mom, Nancy struggles with the feeling that she is not contributing financially to the household. Although her husband has never made her feel guilty or suggested that she is not doing her part, Nancy misses the sense of pride and independence that comes with earning her own income.

Nancy also feels guilty for not giving her daughter Ruby the same level of attention as her son Raymond. Ruby is her "easy kid," and Nancy sometimes takes advantage of her calm and relaxed nature, letting her watch cartoons for long stretches. Ruby "will even put herself down for a nap!" Nancy exclaims. Despite being a peaceful presence in Nancy's life, Ruby still wants to be acknowledged and reminds Nancy that she needs special attention too. Sometimes, when Nancy is changing Raymond's medical equipment, Ruby will show signs of jealousy, explaining that she deserves to have devices on her body too.

Now that Raymond is in school for part of the day, Nancy has some one-on-one time with Ruby, which they both enjoy. While putting Ruby in daycare could provide both mother and daughter with extra opportunities for socialization and entertainment, it would also mean working full-time just to pay for those services. For now, Nancy has decided that the trade-off isn't worth it. In Nancy's vision of a perfect future, she would be able to work from home, giving her the comfort of being there as needed for both kids, while still being able to contribute to the family income. Nancy also has a good deal of experience working in fabric and craft stores and would like to return at least part-time to that environment. As many stay-at-home moms can relate to, sometimes she just misses the adult interaction that comes from working outside the home.

Although Nancy's movements aren't restricted by a job, her ability to get around during the day is limited because they are a one-car family and that car is often on the road with her husband. Raymond has to take two separate buses to get to and from school each day, and the one, to one-and-a-half hour commute, can be stressful for Nancy. Nancy points out that the bus monitors are highly attentive and make sure that Raymond has all of his equipment with him before pulling away from the curb. They always check not only his seatbelt, but his glucose monitor, to make sure that he is set up for a safe ride home. Despite these precautions, the fact that Nancy cannot reach Raymond for extended periods in case of an emergency remains a persistent source of stress for her. The distance and lack of immediate access to her son creates a constant worry. To mitigate the risk of an urgent low blood sugar when Raymond is away from home, Nancy tends to let Raymond's blood sugar run a bit higher than she would like during the school day. As a result, his A1C isn't exactly where she'd like it to be, but for now, "it's just one of those things."

To alleviate Nancy's worries, she finds solace in the fact that Raymond loves school and eagerly boards the bus each day. He is delighted to attend parties and social events with his classmates, and the mothers in their social circle have been incredibly supportive in making sure Raymond never feels left out. Recently, a classmate's mother even reached out to discuss gluten-free meal options for an upcoming event, a gesture that deeply touched Nancy. Despite the challenges posed by Raymond's diabetes, developmental complications, and celiac, Nancy is grateful for the kindness and understanding shown by those in their social network.In spite of everyone's best efforts, accidental gluten exposure is a frequent occurrence for young children with celiac. It can result from cross-contamination on shared food surfaces or from a child's curiosity to try tempting foods on the "forbidden list". When Raymond is exposed to gluten, he often becomes ill for several days. Unfortunately, he struggles to communicate his discomfort due to his verbal delays. To reduce the risk of gluten exposure, Nancy tries to have gluten-free "duplicates" of the treats Raymond may encounter when they are out, but this isn't always possible. The challenge of managing gluten exposure is a constant reminder of the difficulties that come with managing celiac disease with young ones.

To make mealtime manageable, Nancy serves gluten-free dishes to both children, even though this means a more expensive grocery bill. During lunch, when Raymond is at school, Nancy may give Ruby a sandwich made with regular bread, but for dinner when both kids are together, the entire meal must be gluten-free. This not only reduces the risk of cross-contamination but also gives Nancy a break from intense supervision. She finds that the kids tend to eat better when she isn't constantly watching over them and they enjoy sharing food from each other's plates. This is one way Nancy has found to give herself a little break in the evening when she doesn't have a co-parent to relieve her. Finding these types of "life hacks" early on can help parents maintain their own mental health when caring for young children with complex medical needs.

Of course, celiac isn't the only condition that complicates Raymond's diabetes management. Handling medical procedures like insulin shots and device changes can be a challenge for children with complex medical needs, especially when they are neurodiverse like Raymond. While prepping kids with a simple "you have 3 minutes to play before we change your Dex," might work in some instances, in the midst of unexpected events, like nighttime device failures, advanced preparation techniques may not always be an option. Fortunately for Nancy, Raymond still responds well to reward systems and takes great enjoyment from getting new device stickers. Raymond is especially fond of holiday-themed stickers like candy-corn adhesive patches around Halloween. Of course, Ruby likes to get in on the fun too, so Nancy was excited when a woman who she heard interviewed on her favorite JuiceBox podcast offered to send her some extra Pod stickers. She points out that Etsy is also a great place to find good deals on decorative adhesive multi-packs.

Although Nancy is finding her groove, she admits that sometimes the challenges of raising a young child with complex medical issues while also tending full-time to the needs of a toddler gets the better of her. She points out that she often passes out completely when in the dentist's chair because it's one of the most relaxing places for her to be. Recently she fell and broke her ankle. She actually had walked around with that injury for days before her husband got home and encouraged her to see a doctor. As she points out, taking that time to tend to her own medical needs wasn't an option until that point because "I still had to make lunch and get Raymond on the bus." She noted that getting her bone set was the "most relaxed" she had been that entire day.

"I just can't afford to get sick" she says. I'm sure many reading this story can relate.

Briana Dean and Ford: Diabetes Management: A Family Affair

To stay consistent with the style of the other stories in this book, I'll be sharing Briana's perspective on the experiences of her family with diabetes. However, after hearing Briana's story, I realized that it would be unfair to present it as just another mother's tale. Unlike the other mothers I've talked to over the years, Briana was not the main caregiver for her son Ford during his younger years. Instead, that responsibility fell on her husband Dean. So, while this story will be told through Briana's eyes, I will make sure to give due recognition to Dean's remarkable role in providing full-time care for a toddler with diabetes.

To bring out each mother's story, I often go through her old Facebook posts, blogs, and other collections of memories and pictures. This helps me revive some of the thoughts and experiences that may have been forgotten and not shared during the interview process. When I went through Briana's social media updates from 2011, I stumbled upon an anniversary post celebrating 12 years of marriage with her husband Dean. In the post, she wrote, "I'm lucky to have such a wonderful husband and I'm looking forward to many more great years together!"

While many people express similar sentiments about their partners on anniversaries, in talking with Briana, I could sense how genuinely she felt those words then and still does today, 12 years later. Above all, Briana exudes an immense sense of gratitude for the sacrifices her husband Dean has made for the family. After the birth of Ford in August 2008, Briana took a brief maternity leave of just 6 weeks. To support Briana's career and ensure Ford could receive care at home, Dean agreed to be the stay-at-home parent. Though Dean eventually returned to part-time work in 2019, a lot transpired in those years.

Briana first opened up about her story with me in April of 2017, seven years after Ford's diabetes diagnosis. She was already a seasoned caregiver and was eager to share her insights with others. Like many other participants in this project, Briana was hopeful that her knowledge could provide comfort and guidance to future parents who may feel overwhelmed by the new and unfamiliar responsibilities that come with caring for a young diabetic. She wanted to help ease their fears, especially for those who may have limited medical experience.

At the time, I had been toying with including a chapter on "Tips and Tricks" that Briana was eager to contribute to. In response to my request for ideas, she shared the following insights:

Briana's Tips & Tricks

1. "My biggest wish I would have known was that 15g of fast-acting is often way too much to treat a low for a toddler. We were constantly rebounding! 4-6 grams was often enough to safely treat a low without a rebound high."

2. "I also wish I had thought to pre-draw syringes (he mostly took .5 or 1 unit at a time) for caregivers. My mother-in-law had trouble seeing the lines. We eventually pre-drew syringes and put them in ziplock bags labeled 1/2 unit and 1 unit. Made it so much easier for her!

3. "My husband said he wished he would have known 'that this would all work out - it's not as dire as it seems'."

Briana's Tips & Tricks Continued

4. "And my mother-in-law said she wished she would have said something earlier when she saw his symptoms; that she could get over her fear of giving him shots."

5. "Also, don't be afraid to ask for help and train someone else. You need to find time for yourself/significant other."

These are all powerful words of wisdom. Honestly, I wish someone had shared them with me when I first started on this journey. Now, nearly 10 years in, I can attest that YES, 15 grams of carbs is A LOT for a toddler! And YES, pre-drawing syringes is a great strategy--especially when mixing long and fast-acting insulins or asking for help from caregivers who might have vision impairments. And YES, YES, YES--train others and ask for help whenever possible. Caregiver fatigue is real and generally best to avoid in the first place. I truly hope that Briana's insights help those who follow in her footsteps to avoid some of the mistakes that she and I both made in the early days.

Unfortunately, after a series of moves and new beginnings, I lost touch with Briana and our interactions became limited to occasional support board conversations. However, when I recently put out a call for new submissions, Briana kindly agreed to revisit her story, eight years after our initial connection. I am truly grateful for this time-lapse as our chat felt like catching up with an old friend. We had a good laugh about how much our lives had changed over the years, with Briana chuckling, "Remember when you had to be within 10 feet of the CGM, and there was no remote monitoring?"

In reflecting on how much of our conversation was, “remember the old days when...”, I could imagine “Dr. Rick” (The Progressive Insurance guy) popping in and pointing out that he couldn't "save [us] from becoming [our] parents," but that he could save us a ton of money if we bundled our home and car insurance. I wonder if Briana would be interested in such an arrangement.

But joking aside, during my conversation with Briana, I realized how little I actually knew about Ford's story. Our initial connection was mostly through Facebook Messenger chats; we never had a chance to have an in-depth interview. As a result, so much was missing from the initial picture. What follows is a wide-lens look at how this family's journey unfolded over the course of twelve years.

On March 8th, 2011, Briana shared her excitement on Facebook with her friends and family, announcing that she had signed Ford up for swimming lessons and that he was set to start on March 20th. However, the celebratory mood was short-lived as the family received the devastating news the very next day that Ford had been diagnosed with Type 1 diabetes. This meant that Briana and Dean were faced with a new set of difficult decisions around Ford's care.

Briana had aspirations of going back to school to earn her bachelor's degree, but this would require long work days followed by nights spent studying and completing coursework. This meant the new medical responsibilities would fall on Dean's shoulders. Despite the added challenge, Dean eagerly accepted and in June of 2011, Briana became a full-time working and student mom, buoyed by the love and support of her husband.

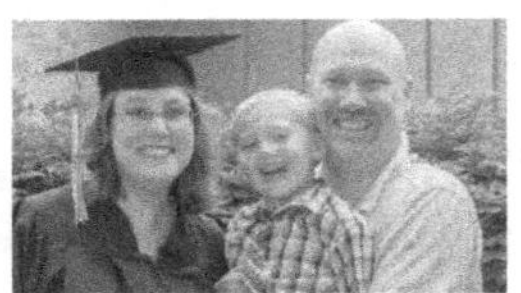

This picture is a screenshot from an interview that Briana did with Walsh College, following her graduation. It is titled "When There's a Will, There's a Way: Balancing Life and School at Walsh College" and can be found on YouTube.

In recounting the early years of managing life with Type 1, Briana shared how much time and energy Dean had sacrificed to keep their newly diagnosed toddler safe. In the fall of 2012, they decided to put Ford into preschool, but as many parents quickly find out, placing a young diabetic child in a daycare or preschool setting can be more work than keeping them home. Every time a device fails or blood sugars becomes stubbornly high or low, a parent must drop what they are doing and race back to make things right. "We would drop him off with his blood sugar at 180 and he would nosedive to 115 double-arrows down [a reference to the trend readings on the continuous glucose monitor]. So my husband would stay at preschool the entire time and do his work there. The teachers used to joke that they should have him on the payroll."

They continued to make things work like this for two years, but, "Eventually, we just decided to homeschool," explained Briana. "We discussed sending Ford to public school for kindergarten in the fall, but my husband, Dean, and I agreed that even if he went, Dean likely wouldn't be able to go back to work because we would need child care during the summer/breaks and the ability to get to the school at the drop of a hat. So we figured if he was going to continue staying home, it might be easier to homeschool Ford."

In the diabetes community, discussions around homeschooling are a frequent topic of conversation. Parents are torn between the difficulties of sending a young child out into the world without proper self-care skills and the challenges of staying at home full-time. The financial impact of lost wages, the challenge of providing enough social activities, and the ability to deliver a proper education are all concerns that weigh heavily on parents. Usually, it's the mother who takes on the role of full-time teacher, but in Briana and Dean's case, it was Dean who made the sacrifice. He continued to delay career plans to take on the rewarding but unpaid job of homeschooling Ford.

As Ford approached middle school, he longed for the social experiences of a traditional school day. The family made plans for him to start 6th grade at a local brick-and-mortar school, but in the spring of 2020, Covid took the world by storm, and they decided to hold off. Finally, last spring, in April of 2022, Ford entered middle school as a 7th grader, using the last quarter of the school year as a trial run. To increase their chances of success, Briana worked with the school to establish a 504 Plan for Ford (an educational support plan that helps spell out the specific accommodations needed to allow a child with a disability to access their education).

~ A Note From Erin ~

For parents of school-aged diabetics, having a 504 Plan in place can provide peace of mind and ensure their child can manage medical needs at school without obstacles. The plan outlines crucial accommodations, such as being able to use a phone for glucose monitoring, unrestricted access to water and restrooms, alternative settings for glucose management, and extra time for tests and assignments if blood sugar imbalances affect academic progress. Without a 504 Plan, children with diabetes may encounter resistance from teachers or be excluded from certain school activities, which is illegal.

~ Erin's Note Continued ~

Without a plan and understanding of ADA protections, some well-meaning teachers and administrators may accidentally violate a student's rights. For families of children with disabilities, including those with diabetes, it's important to know that student rights are protected by federal guidelines. The Individuals with Disabilities Education Act (IDEA) and the Americans with Disabilities Act (ADA) ensure that schools and daycare centers cannot discriminate against children with disabilities. Although the interpretation and implementation of these laws may vary by state, there is plenty of information available to parents.

A simple internet search can bring up valuable resources, including sites run by organizations such as JDRF and the American Diabetes Association. If parents encounter resistance in establishing a support plan for their child, online forums can be a great place to turn for help. With members from all 50 states, these communities offer a wealth of tips, tricks, and insights tailored to specific locations.

This project was born with the aim of sharing the experiences of families with infants and toddlers living with diabetes, but it has evolved into so much more. It's a resource where parents can gain the information and courage they need to be strong advocates for themselves and their children in situations where they may have felt vulnerable in the past. Initially, the focus was on the stories of infants and toddlers, and the complexities of 504 plans and IEPs (Individualized Education Plans) were not part of the discussion.

~ Erin's Note Continued ~

After being part of online forums for nearly a decade, I've seen a growing number of parents seeking help for their 3 and 4-year-olds who are having trouble finding daycares or preschools that can accommodate their children's needs. By sharing Briana and Ford's journey over the course of 12 years, this project offers valuable insights into the world of diabetes management and the challenges that come with it.

~ End Erin's Note ~

Being the parent of a child with Type 1 diabetes comes with its own set of challenges, beyond just the logistical and legal hurdles. As Briana mentioned in our conversation, supporting her son Ford's mental well-being is just as important as supporting his physical health. This includes finding the right balance between arranging professional therapy sessions and following Ford's lead on important decisions, as well as encouraging positive social interactions and avoiding toxic relationships--even when those relationships involve family members.

During my conversation with Briana, she shared some of the difficulties her family faced after Ford was diagnosed with celiac disease at the age of 5. For children like Ford who have to manage multiple diagnoses, the challenges of celiac can be even harder to handle than diabetes. Unlike diabetes, where you can eat anything as long as you balance it with insulin, with celiac, you have to always be mindful of what you eat to avoid gluten exposure. Despite the increasing availability of gluten-free options, it can still be difficult to find safe food in some settings. For someone with celiac disease, eating away from home can be a challenge as the person either has to bring their own food, go without eating, or take the risk of experiencing complications from gluten exposure. According to Briana, Ford frequently expresses frustration living with this added burden of life with celiac. He tells her, "I just want to be able to open a cabinet and eat without thinking about it."

For many children with celiac, ingesting gluten can lead to severe abdominal pain. For those who also have diabetes, gluten exposure can result in persistent low blood sugar levels as their inflamed gut struggles to absorb nutrients properly, making the management of the two diseases together even more complicated. In the weeks leading up to Ford's celiac diagnosis, they found night-time blood sugar management especially complicated. "One really scary night, we gave him juice right before bed. His blood sugar was 90 with the arrow on the monitor straight across." For those unfamiliar with continuous glucose monitors, an arrow straight across is usually a welcome sign as it means steady numbers that aren't likely to shift dramatically up or down any time soon. On this particular night, they were trying to get Ford's blood sugar up over 100 to avoid some of the middle-of-the-night drops they had been experiencing at the time.

Unfortunately, even after giving over 100 ounces of juice (which is typically a lot for someone with diabetes), they still couldn't get his blood sugar to go up over 100. Ford was terrified to go to sleep and asked his mom, "What happens if my number goes to zero." Within a week of this episode, they decided to have a "scope" (or upper endoscopy) done and confirmed the secondary diagnosis of celiac.

Briana recounted how family gatherings became a source of emotional pain for Ford following his celiac diagnosis. Family members would "gush" about all the delicious gluten-filled food and treats, while pointing Ford to a separate section of gluten-free options saying, "Oh, that's the stuff for you." While their intentions might have been good, this kind of reminder of what he couldn't eat and how different he was from everyone else was especially tough for five-year-old Ford. Eventually, the family stopped attending gatherings altogether. As Briana shared, sometimes you just have to "find the people who are going to support you and they become your family."

According to Briana, she tries her best not to restrict Ford's diet more than is necessary. When he was going through a phase of eating cereal for breakfast every morning, she tried to go along with it, as most kids love cereal. However, they were struggling with post-meal blood sugar spikes, so she worked with Ford to understand the benefits of limiting his cereal intake. Briana explains, "I don't want to restrict him because I know he'll have to make independent eating choices in the future," but she also recognized that as a parent, sometimes she would need to step in and show him how certain food choices he was making could be self-sabotaging.

Throughout Ford's different dietary phases, such as being a vegetarian or following a high-protein diet, Briana has supported him while continuing to educate him on making healthy choices. With high-carb meals like cereal, she has gotten a little more firm, limiting his cereal intake to weekends when blood sugar spikes won't impact his performance in school. She knows that managing his diabetes and celiac disease is a constant balancing act, but she is dedicated to supporting Ford in every way she can.

Ford and his family have been lucky to have care providers who have first-hand experience with conditions like diabetes and celiac. For example, the school district nurse who helped create Ford's 504 plan also has celiac and was able to advocate for Ford's needs. When the school principal suggested serving gluten-free meals in the regular cafeteria, the nurse explained the risk of cross-contamination and pushed for a safer solution. Additionally, Ford has worked with two therapists, both of whom live with diabetes, offering him a sense of connection and understanding that is invaluable for supporting his mental health.

Living with an invisible disease like celiac or diabetes can be isolating for young children, but having care providers who can relate to their struggles is a powerful source of comfort and support. Having someone say, "I understand because I have this too," can be incredibly valuable for boosting the mental well-being of kids with these conditions. Ford and his family have been extremely fortunate to have such resources.

One of the reasons Ford's family sought out mental health support was that they started noticing Ford's struggles with memory and focus. While there is some research exploring the prevalence of ADHD in children with diabetes and its impact on blood sugar control, this is outside the scope of this book. Anecdotally, however, after a series of assessments, Ford was diagnosed with ADHD, anxiety, and OCD, and he found that taking medication to treat these conditions has greatly improved his overall well-being. Unlike his physical conditions of celiac and diabetes, Ford doesn't seem to have the same resentment towards his mental health differences. Although he was resistant to adding additional medication to his routine at first, now that he sees how much he benefits from it, he welcomes the relief that comes from taking a daily pill.

Briana shares that "as disgruntled as he is with his multiple conditions, Ford is very open about them." Overall, Ford has become more open about discussing his conditions with others. Briana shares that "he likes to tell people that he's a cyborg. He likes that it throws people off." He also finds it funny to make comments in public about "being high," and watching for quizzical looks from strangers. Recently, his classmates gifted him the nickname of "Beep Beep". Briana and Ford don't know if that's in response to the fact that he is named after a car or because his medical devices often "beep" alerts throughout the day--maybe it's a little bit of both. Either way, Ford seems to be comfortable with the new term of endearment. Despite his multiple conditions, Ford has a positive attitude and a sense of humor about his experiences. His openness and willingness to talk about his conditions serve as a reminder of the importance of mental health support for children with chronic conditions.

Briana's main focus now is empowering Ford to become more self-sufficient in managing his care. She encourages him to take an active role in filling out medical paperwork and communicating directly with his doctor during endocrinology appointments. This can be a significant and sometimes frightening milestone for parents who have been caring for their child's diabetes from a young age.

Teaching a child to independently manage physical aspects of care, such as changing continuous glucose monitors (CGMs) and insulin sites, can also be a challenge. When a parent has always performed these tasks with both hands, it can be difficult to teach a young person to do so on their own, often using only one hand, such as when attaching a device to an arm. For years, Ford has worn his insulin pump and continuous glucose monitor attached to his upper buttock, as it was the only part of his thin body that had enough tissue to accommodate the devices. However, this location can be difficult for a child to reach and apply the devices on their own. With the area now covered in scar tissue from years of overuse, it's a good time for Ford to learn how to apply devices to new parts of his body.

As Briana shares, she was aware that consistent use of the same area of Ford's body for his pump and CGM would eventually result in the development of scar tissue. However, she was willing to "use up" this space while Ford was young to preserve other areas, such as his upper arms and legs, for when he was ready to transition to self-management in later years. Briana is not forcing independence and is trying to allow Ford to assume responsibility at his own pace, but she is committed to helping Ford gain the independence and confidence he needs to manage his own health.

Footnote: As the former Student Services Coordinator (running the special education department) for a local elementary school, I have quite a bit of information to share on this subject as well and am all too happy to share what I know directly with parents. Although I don't want to derail Briana and Ford's story any further on this subject, I feel the need to emphasize that I am more than happy to serve as a direct resource on this subject for those who are feeling lost. Reaching out to me directly through social media channels or my website (as of this writing ConfessionsOfAnAcad emicMom.Com) will not be viewed as rude or intrusive.

Wendy & Liam: The Challenges of Life with Multiple Complex Disabilities

Wendy and Liam's story is by far the most complex of all the families captured in this book. When Liam was first diagnosed with diabetes, he was already living with several complicated conditions, including epilepsy, cerebral palsy, mild but unilateral hearing loss and gastroparesis. As the years have progressed, his hearing loss has become profound and he has been diagnosed as functionally nonverbal. At the time of this writing, Wendy and Liam are in ongoing assessment for ADHD, speech Apraxia and autism. While I will touch on some of these conditions throughout their story and highlight the ways in which living with multiple conditions can complicate diabetes management, I will make every effort to concentrate the focus on life with Type 1 Diabetes. Wendy describes the tale of Liam's diagnosis as "harrowing": "We went in for his g-tube surgery right at age 2 in August of 2016. Unbeknownst to me, the major children's hospital that was performing the surgery missed that his FASTING BG was 140. About 2-3 weeks later we were in Nashville for a special therapy we do for him (Anat Baniel Method); and he went into DKA and had to be admitted to the PICU at Vandy."

In looking back on pictures from that August it is hard to believe that this was a child about to be diagnosed with diabetes. He had the cute chubby leg rolls of a well-fed baby, and can be seen laughing and giggling while playing with one of the family dogs--a beautiful white and tan collie. On September 5, Liam returned following a successful recovery from his GI-Tube surgery. Wendy was happy to report that Liam was "doing pretty well adjusting to his new status as a Tubie baby" and that he seemed "much more alert and more controlled with his movements", which she attributed to the more effective administration of nutritional formula and changed dosaging with his seizure medicine.

On Facebook, Wendy showed off a thriving Liam, sporting rosy cheeks and a new denim newsboy cap. It seemed as if the worst was behind them. Until just two short weeks later when Liam started showing signs of medical distress. Wendy and her husband rushed Liam back to the hospital, only to find that his blood sugar was highly elevated and he was in DKA.

Wendy expressed some frustration over how all of this played out. Had the doctors run repeated blood sugar tests during the time Liam was in the hospital for his G-tube surgery, this crisis episode could have been averted. But with all the other complicating factors being managed for Liam, it seems his irregular blood glucose was overlooked.

Fortunately, Liam's hospital stay was relatively short, and by September 21, they were on their way back home again, with a big smile on Liam's face and his blue eyes sparkling against the turquoise stripes of his little onsie. By this time, the Williams family was well accustomed to managing obstacles. Diabetes was just one more condition they would figure out how to bring into the fold.

Because Liam was on a combination of breastmilk and tube feedings at the time of diagnosis, special considerations had to be made regarding delivery of insulin and carb counting. Wendy was especially worried about the possibility of the GI Tube being accidentally ripped out after giving insulin, but the doctors seemed to dismiss her fears. They told her that in the unlikely event that the GI Tube gets detached during a feeding, she should simply give glucagon to compensate for the loss of carbs.

Unfortunately, it didn't take long for Wendy to face this fear head-on. Just two weeks after diagnosis, Liam's feeding tube was dislodged shortly after insulin had been administered. They piled into the car and rushed off to the emergency room, with Wendy at the wheel. "I was going 90 MPH on the interstate when we came to a mile-long pile-up. I raced up onto the shoulder, dodging signs as I went."

As Wendy attempted to navigate the emergency lane, her husband worked to continuously monitor Liam's blood sugar through a series of finger checks. He struggled to prepare the life-saving glucagon solution, but couldn't manage the task as the car raced and bumped along. Wendy eventually pulled over so that glucagon could be administered and they could transfer Liam to the ambulance that had met them along the way.

When they arrived at the hospital, the medical team had to force-dilate Liam's stoma so that the g-tube could be reinserted. According to some basic research through Google, the stoma (through which the GI-tube is inserted) can take weeks to fully close, but it will start closing and healing itself within a few hours of tube removal. In Liam's case, the stoma had already started to close by the time they reached the hospital.

Liam was also still breastfeeding at this time, so as Wendy explains, "We had to navigate vomiting and the g tube and the breastfeeding and all the varying absorption rates with the Gastroparesis." Wendy often tried to combine feedings (feeding through the g-tube while also nursing) but special care had to be taken to minimize the risk of removing the g-tube accidentally. She often used a ring-sling to keep him tight to her body and reduce the risks associated with too many moving parts around medical tubing, but even with her best efforts, that first time the tube came out would not be the last.

By Septemer 23, just two weeks after Liam's release from the hospital, Wendy was reminding people of the importance of voting, and by the end of that same month, she was sharing medical research news about everything from the artificial pancreas to defibrillator drones. It was back to business as usual!

Within two months, they were able to get Liam on a continuous glucose monitor (the Dexcom) and within about 6 months, they were able to get him going on a tubeless insulin pump (the Omnipod). This isn't to say that things were easy. As most parents who manage Type 1 in young diabetics will attest, technology is both a blessing and a curse. Although the technology makes life more manageable when it is working smoothly, technology often fails, creating more chaos than traditional management techniques could have ever done--It sure would have been helpful to have a continuous monitor alert to Liam's rapidly increasing blood sugar after the GI pump delivered a double dose of formula, but that was still a few weeks away.

At the end of October, Wendy and Liam found themselves back in the hospital--this time as the result of regular toddler shenanigans rather than the consequence of medical complications. Liam had been playing with one of his favorite toys when he face-planted right onto it, giving himself a fairly deep gash across the forehead. After a quick stint in the ER to ensure that he was OK, Wendy happily reported to friends and family that "He is home and shaking his booty to some music!" And so continued their journey of ups and downs in the life of a family with a medically complex toddler.

In November, just two months after his initial diagnosis, the Williams family excitedly unpacked their first shipment of Dexcom receivers. Wendy carefully applied the sensor/transmitter combination for the first time, while Liam's daddy held him carefully in his arms. Liam shed a few quick tears, but quickly went back to bouncing at the side of his new trainset, again marking a new phase in their journey.

March was a turbulent month, marked by thunderstorms, tornadoes and insulin pump failures. But on March 29, Liam was treated to a day at the park for the first time since his diabetes diagnosis. Wendy remembers that "Liam loved it so much and did not want to stop swinging. He enjoyed the wind in his hair and watching his shadow swing with him as well as watching the other children." They eventually had to go home to help Liam cool off and get his tube feeding and he cried the entire car trip home. Wendy vowed to make trips to the park a more regular part of their routine.

When Liam was one year old (about nine months prior to Liam's diabetes diagnosis), Wendy made the difficult decision to quit the job she loved, working at a university, so that she could stay home and focus on Liam's medical needs. Although Wendy is grateful to have had the opportunity to do that for her son, becoming a full-time stay-at-home mom and caregiver for a medically complex child meant sacrificing opportunities for self-care and independent activities. As Liam approached his third birthday, Wendy started finding ways to reintroduce "grownup" time into her life, taking time to eat lunch out by herself on occasion and going back to the gym. Getting Liam into some Early Intervention programs turned out to be a blessing for them both.

By this time in their journey, Liam's hearing loss had evolved to "profound," so Wendy started working on getting him into a local school for deaf children. Unfortunately, his diabetes became a complicating factor that was used to bar him from admission. Wendy had to fight for three years to get him admitted to the school. In that time, she taught herself (and Liam) ASL and created a few new signs for diabetes and g-tube related communication. She also made tutorial videos related to g-tube insertion and specialized nursing holds for children with physical impairments. Wendy considers herself not just an advocate for Liam, but for the entire community of those managing multiple medically complex conditions.

One of the fights that Wendy has taken on is trying to get Liam into the special "Katie Beckett" Medicaid program. This particular Medicaid plan is specially funded through the federal government to address the needs of minor children living with complex medical conditions. The goal of the program is to allow such individuals to live and receive treatment at home as opposed to institutionalized care. What distinguishes this type of Medicaid from others is that families that might typically be excluded (due to family income or health insurance status) can still be eligible. Of course, this all sounds easier on paper than most people experience in reality. In 2019, after months of working toward getting Liam approved for Katie Beckett funding, the program director called to let Wendy know that if they opted for this coverage, Liam would likely have to drop his CHIP insurance.

Wendy was devastated. When she first messaged me about the news, she was still awaiting a final decision, hopeful that common sense would prevail. If those with private insurance and higher family incomes can qualify for Katie Beckett funding, those in lower income brackets, and accessing CHIP certainly shouldn't be disqualified. But as every parent of a child with disabilities can attest, the quest for medical coverage is an ongoing battle.

As Wendy says, "Suffice it to say I will never stop fighting and pushing for the latest and best care and methods for him. I even got trained in Reiki to use energy healing with him." She has also fought for access to a wide variety of therapies, including music therapy, the Anat Baniel Method (a neuroplasticity/NeuroMovement therapy), Hippotherapy, Aquatherapy, PT, OT, Speech, and feeding therapy. If there is a technique out there to be tried and which offers the possibility of improving quality of life for Liam, Wendy will find a way to access it!

Of course, there's more to medical management than professional therapeutics. As Wendy emphasizes, finding the right nutritional balance for Liam is critical in managing all of his medical needs. Unfortunately, this isn't always so easy for a child who needs to be tube-fed. "Amazingly the professional medical community at large is woefully ignorant of nutrition and has fought the switch to real blended food for a long time," Wendy explains. "The major companies are starting to get more on board because patients and families have said 'hell no, we need real food. But it is hard to trust companies like Nestle to be sure to have a truly healthy product when they have knowingly been harming the health of patients for decades." Wendy feels that "Liam's Gastroparesis has gotten progressively better with dietary changes and that Whole Story Meals works the best for him." She has also incorporated probiotics and digestive enzymes into his daily regimen to help enhance nutritional absorption.

Now that Liam is a little older, she is working on adding more oral feedings into his diet. As any parent who has made this transition from liquid diet (breastmilk and/or formula) to solids can attest, the introduction of new foods automatically adds a new layer of complexity to glucose management. As Wendy points out, access to an insulin pump (especially a closed-loop system as Liam has) is invaluable when trying to manage such transitions. It can allow for fine-tuning of insulin delivery in response to fluctuating blood sugars.

As most parents of young type-1 children find, being able to adjust basal rates is key to tackling blood sugar fluctuations in response to the intake surprises that are common with young diabetics. For example, when a little one sneaks into some snacks that weren't planned for, an increased basal rate in combination with a bolus to cover the estimated carbs consumed (one can't always be sure of what was actually eaten) is a helpful way to cover carbs with insulin quickly, while also leaving an "escape plan" in case blood sugar starts to drop too quickly. Unlike with long-lasting insulin (which can't be removed from the body once administered), basal rates can be turned down in response to suddenly dropping numbers. This is also extremely useful for kids with comorbid conditions like Liam's gastroparesis or Connor's celiac, which often interfere with nutrient absorption.

As Wendy points out, despite all of his medical conditions, Liam is very much like any other young child. He gets moody and throws temper tantrums when frustrated or overtired, but he also has preferences, interests and joys like everyone else. According to his mom, "some of Liam's favorite things are dogs and wolves." He also loves music (especially his favorite band, Coldplay and hearing his mom sing, "which sometimes makes him emotional"). He gets super excited while jumping on the trampoline--who doesn't?! And loves Disney movies. One of his favorite pastimes is acting out scenes from his favorite shows and movies.

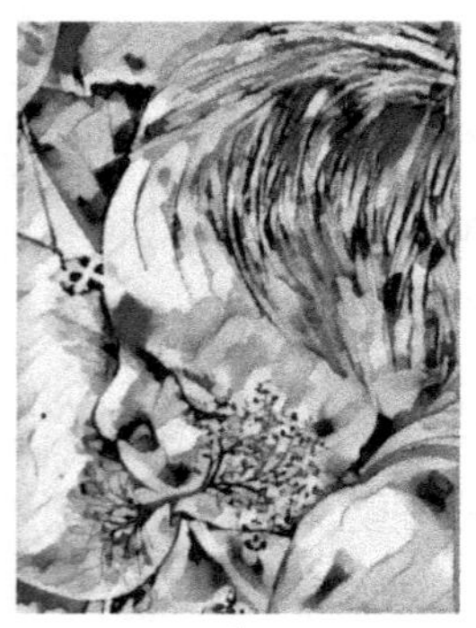

A watercolor print that Wendy created from a photograph of her nursing Liam after the trauma of that initial g-tube experience

As much joy as Liam brings to his family, the management of so many complex factors has resulted in increased family tension. According to Calleen Petersen's (2018) review of a longitudinal study related to divorce rates for parents of children with special needs, the risk for divorce is not inherently higher for this demographic, but with increased stress comes increased challenges. While parents who find themselves with a newly diagnosed child should not assume their marriage to be "doomed", they should recognize that staying together might take a bit of extra work and attention.

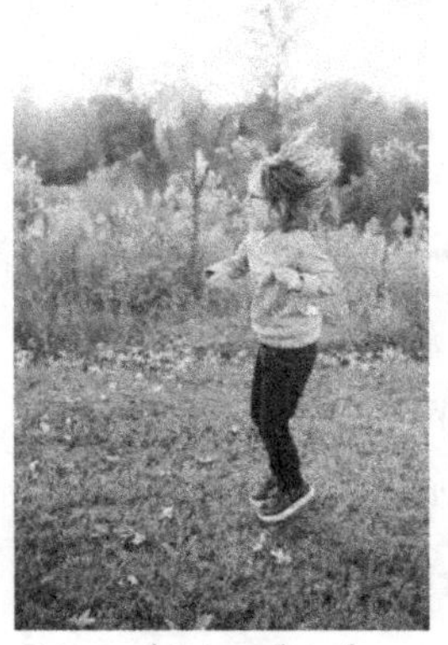

Liam living his best life and doing one of the things he loves most in the world--jumping!

Unfortunately for Wendy, she is likely approaching another period of "changing family dynamics" as related to the stress of parenting a child with complex medical needs. But she has proven herself to be quite strong and resilient, so I remain optimistic that she will continue to live a full and happy life with her children, continuously celebrating all of the wonderful little milestones that present themselves along the way.

~ A Final Note From Erin ~

Thank you so much for reading this book! I really hope you enjoyed it and found it helpful. If you have a moment, I would be incredibly grateful if you could leave a review at your favorite book retailer's online site. Whether it's a simple "Loved it" or "Not for me," your feedback means the world to me. Every review helps other readers find this powerful chronicle and can make a real difference for independent authors like me. Thank you for your support and for being a part of this community of resilience, bravery, and love.

I'd also like to thank all my amazing beta readers and pre-release reviewers! Your feedback has been invaluable. If you're interested in joining my beta team and getting early access to my upcoming projects, please visit my website at ConfessionsOfAnAcademicMom and leave a comment so I can add you to the team. I look forward to connecting with you!

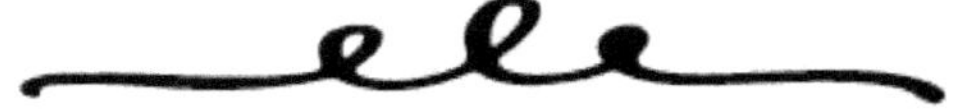

Glossary

The following is a list of medical or technical terms and definitions (in alphabetical order) that relate to the stories shared in this book. They are primarily focused on diabetes and celiac, but other conditions mentioned in the stories will be defined here as well.

Note: No reference will be provided for the following descriptions as they are a conglomerate of information readily available on the internet. The definitions, as written, have been created with the help of the artificial intelligence software known as ChatGPT.

504 Plan:

A 504 Plan is a plan created to support children with disabilities in the classroom. It outlines the accommodations and support that a child with a disability, such as diabetes, needs in order to have equal access to education. The plan is named after Section 504 of the Rehabilitation Act of 1973, which prohibits discrimination based on disability.

In the case of school-aged children with diabetes, a 504 Plan can help minimize the risk of discrimination and alienation during school activities. It can ensure that the child has access to necessary equipment and supplies, such as insulin and glucose monitoring devices, and that the school staff is trained in how to use them in case of an emergency. The plan can also specify the times and locations where the child can check their blood glucose levels and receive insulin injections, as well as ensure that the child is able to eat at the appropriate times and have access to snacks and meals that are in line with their diabetes management plan.

By having a 504 Plan in place, school-aged children with diabetes can feel supported and included in their school community, and their diabetes management can be better integrated into their school day. This can help reduce stress and anxiety for both the child and their caregivers, and improve their overall health and well-being.

A1C:

A1C refers to a blood test that provides an average of a person's blood glucose levels over the past 2-3 months. It is commonly used to monitor the effectiveness of diabetes management and track progress over time. A1C levels reflect the amount of hemoglobin in the blood that has glucose molecules attached to it, and a higher level of hemoglobin A1C indicates higher blood glucose levels.

For people with diabetes, monitoring A1C levels is crucial as it provides insight into their overall blood glucose control. Poor glucose control can result in a number of serious health problems, including diabetic complications such as heart disease, nerve damage, and kidney disease. An A1C test provides a more comprehensive view of blood glucose control than a single blood glucose test and can help identify trends and patterns in a person's blood glucose levels.

The American Diabetes Association recommends that people with diabetes aim for an A1C level of 7% or lower. However, the target A1C level can vary depending on factors such as age, overall health, and the presence of other medical conditions. A healthcare provider can help determine the appropriate target A1C level for each individual. Regular monitoring of A1C levels, in combination with regular monitoring of blood glucose levels and lifestyle adjustments, can help people with diabetes maintain good glucose control and reduce the risk of complications.

ADD/ADHD, or Attention Deficit [Hyperactivity] Disorder:

ADD/ADHD is a neurodevelopmental disorder characterized by inattention and impulsiveness and can present with or without hyperactivity. While not directly related to diabetes, some individuals with diabetes find that managing their symptoms of ADD/ADHD can help them better control their blood glucose levels. This may be due to improved focus and organization, leading to better adherence to a diabetic management plan. Additionally, individuals with ADD/ADHD who have difficulty following through on tasks related to diabetes care may benefit from structure and routine provided by treatment for their condition.

There is some evidence to suggest a correlation between diabetes and ADHD. Research suggests that individuals with uncontrolled diabetes may have a higher risk of developing ADHD or similar symptoms. On the other hand, individuals with ADD/ADHD may be at higher risk of developing type 2 diabetes due to lifestyle factors such as a sedentary lifestyle and/or poor dietary choices. In simple terms, the connection between diabetes and ADHD is not yet fully understood, but there may be a link between the two conditions and it is important for individuals with either condition to receive proper care and treatment to manage their symptoms.

Artificial Pancreas:

An artificial pancreas, also known as an automated insulin delivery system, is a device that aims to mimic the functions of a healthy pancreas by automatically monitoring blood glucose levels and delivering insulin as needed. It is comprised of a continuous glucose monitor (CGM) and an insulin pump that communicate with each other and adjust insulin delivery in real-time.

The development of an artificial pancreas has been ongoing for several years and is currently in various stages of testing and clinical trials. The goal is to create a system that is reliable, safe, and user-friendly for individuals with diabetes. To date, there have been several trials conducted with both adult and pediatric diabetics, with the aim of improving glucose control and reducing the risk of hypoglycemia and hyperglycemia.

The results of these trials have been promising, with many individuals reporting improved glucose control and reduced burden of managing their diabetes. However, more research and testing are needed before an artificial pancreas can be widely available and covered by insurance.

There are currently three stages of development for an artificial pancreas:

Hybrid closed loop systems: This stage involves using a CGM and an insulin pump together, with algorithms that adjust insulin delivery based on the readings from the CGM.

Fully closed loop systems: This stage involves adding a glucose sensor that measures insulin levels and provides feedback to the insulin pump to adjust insulin delivery in real-time.

Predictive closed loop systems: This stage involves incorporating predictive algorithms that can anticipate glucose changes and adjust insulin delivery accordingly.

Autism:

Autism is a neurodevelopmental disorder that affects communication, social interaction, and behavior. It is typically diagnosed in early childhood and is characterized by difficulty with social communication, repetitive behaviors, and restricted interests. There is some evidence to suggest that individuals with type 1 diabetes may have an increased risk of developing autism, although the exact cause of this connection is not yet known.

Managing diabetes in children with autism can be more challenging due to communication difficulties, repetitive behaviors, and resistance to change. Children with autism may have difficulty understanding the reasons for checking their blood glucose levels or taking insulin injections, leading to non-compliance with their diabetes management plan. Additionally, changes in routine or the introduction of new medical equipment or procedures can be difficult for children with autism, leading to stress and anxiety. When first learning to manage my son's diabetes as impacted by celiac, I found support groups dedicated to these overlapping conditions extremely helpful. Similarly, parents who find themselves faced with the challenge of managing diabetes and autism together will likely find parent groups to be invaluable sources of information and support.

BG: Blood glucose levels:

Blood glucose levels refer to the amount of sugar (glucose) present in a person's bloodstream at any given time. Monitoring blood glucose levels is crucial for individuals with diabetes as it helps to regulate insulin levels and maintain overall health.

There are several ways to monitor blood glucose levels on a daily basis, including:

1.Finger-stick blood glucose testing: This is the most common method of monitoring blood glucose levels. It involves using a small device called a glucometer to take a drop of blood from a finger and measure the glucose level in the sample.

2.Continuous Glucose Monitoring (CGM): CGMs are wearable devices that measure glucose levels in real-time and provide continuous updates throughout the day. They use a small sensor that is inserted under the skin and wirelessly transmit data to a receiver or a smartphone app.

3.Interstitial Fluid Testing: This method involves testing the glucose levels in the fluid between the cells (interstitial fluid) instead of the blood. This method is less invasive than finger-stick testing and is becoming increasingly popular as a means of monitoring blood glucose levels.

Regardless of the method chosen, monitoring blood glucose levels on a daily basis is essential for individuals with diabetes to ensure that their glucose levels are within a safe and healthy range. Abnormal levels can lead to serious health consequences if left unchecked, so it is important to be vigilant and proactive about monitoring glucose levels.

Celiac Disease:

Celiac disease is a digestive disorder caused by an immune reaction to gluten, a protein found in wheat, barley, and rye. When someone with celiac consumes gluten, it triggers an immune response that damages the small intestine, leading to difficulty absorbing nutrients from food. This can result in a wide range of symptoms including abdominal pain, bloating, diarrhea, constipation, weight loss, fatigue, anemia, and skin rashes.

In addition to the physical symptoms, celiac can also be emotionally challenging for young children with the condition. People often judge individuals with celiac for wanting to be "trendy" and this can lead to feelings of isolation and frustration. It is important to remember that celiac is a serious medical condition and individuals with celiac must strictly follow a gluten-free diet in order to manage their symptoms and prevent long-term health complications.

People with Type 1 Diabetes are at a higher risk of developing other autoimmune conditions, such as celiac disease. This is because Type 1

Diabetes and celiac are both autoimmune conditions, and it is common for individuals with one autoimmune condition to develop others. For individuals with both Type 1 Diabetes and celiac, managing their blood glucose levels can become even more complicated, as gluten exposure can lead to symptoms such as abdominal pain, bloating, and diarrhea, which can affect blood glucose levels. It is important for individuals with Type 1 Diabetes and celiac to closely monitor their blood glucose levels and work closely with their healthcare team to manage both conditions.

CGM or Continuous Glucose Monitor:

According to Dr. Irl B. Hirsch, the first continuous glucose monitor was approved by the FDA in 1999, but those early devices did not function the way they do now. Early CGMs collected data that could not be seen by the patient. It was only when the individual took their meter to the doctor's office and downloaded the data onto the medical computer that numbers could be interpreted. The first wide-spread "real-time" monitor (which could alert the patient to fluctuating blood glucose levels throughout the day) wasn't introduced until 2004 by Medtronic. In 2012, Dexcom introduced the G4 (which is the CGM that Connor started with) and in 2015, the G5 opened up the opportunity for care-givers to monitor blood sugar from afar. Connor is now on the G6, which connects to his iPhone via bluetooth and then pushes data to family members' phones consistently throughout the day. While the technology is not perfect, the remote monitoring function afforded by G5 and G6 technology has been a true game changer for many living with this disease.

Developmental Delay (DD):

Developmental delay refers to a child's slower than average progress in achieving milestones in physical, cognitive, and social-emotional skills. Children with developmental delays may experience difficulties in areas such as speech and language, motor skills, and social interaction. This can make disease management, including diabetes management, more complicated. For example, a child with developmental delay may have trouble communicating symptoms of hypoglycemia or understanding the importance of self-care practices. This can make it difficult for caregivers to effectively manage their child's health and well-being, leading to increased stress and frustration. In some cases, children with developmental delays may also require additional support and accommodations in order to effectively manage their diabetes, such as modifications to their treatment plan or specialized support services.

DKA/Diabetic Ketoacidosis:

DKA is a serious complication of diabetes that occurs when the body produces high levels of ketones and blood glucose levels become too high. It is commonly associated with high blood glucose levels, but even people with low blood glucose levels can experience DKA if their insulin levels are insufficient. In such cases, the body cannot use glucose for energy, leading to the production of ketones, which can be toxic if not managed properly. In young children, DKA can present a number of symptoms including excessive thirst, frequent urination, abdominal pain, vomiting, confusion, and a sweet or fruity smell on the breath. If left untreated, DKA can lead to serious health complications, including coma, kidney failure, and even death. It is therefore important to monitor both blood glucose levels and insulin levels in children with diabetes to prevent the onset of DKA.

Emergency Action Plan (EAP):

An EAP is a written document that outlines the steps to be taken in the event of a medical emergency related to diabetes management. It is typically developed by the school in collaboration with the child's parents and healthcare team. The purpose of an EAP is to ensure that appropriate and effective action is taken in the event of a medical emergency.

Common components of an EAP for diabetes management in a school setting include:

•Identification of the child with diabetes and their specific medical needs

•Contact information for the child's healthcare team and parent/guardian

•Step-by-step instructions for managing hypoglycemia (low blood glucose) and hyperglycemia (high blood glucose)

•Protocol for administering insulin and glucagon (if applicable)

•Protocol for continuous glucose monitoring (CGM) management

•Guidance for monitoring and responding to symptoms of diabetic ketoacidosis (DKA)

•Clear instructions for what to do in the event of an emergency, including emergency contact information and emergency response procedures

The EAP is an important tool for ensuring the safety and well-being of children with diabetes in the school setting, and it is important for schools to regularly review and update the plan as needed.

Endo/Endocrinologist:

An endocrinologist (referred to by most in the diabetes community as the "Endo") is a medical doctor who specializes in the diagnosis and treatment of conditions related to hormones and the endocrine system. For children with diabetes, an endocrinologist plays a crucial role in managing their condition and ensuring their overall health and well-being.

Typically, children with diabetes are seen by an endocrinologist on a routine basis, often every three to six months. During these appointments, the endocrinologist will assess the child's overall health, review their blood glucose levels and insulin use, and make any necessary adjustments to their treatment plan. They may also perform tests to check for any potential complications related to diabetes, such as kidney or eye problems.

In addition to routine appointments, the endocrinologist will also be available to provide support and guidance as needed, whether that be in response to an emergency or simply to answer questions and provide advice. The endocrinologist will work closely with the child's primary care physician and any other specialists involved in their care to ensure that they receive the most comprehensive and effective treatment possible.

EoE: Eosinophilic Esophagitis:

EoE is a condition characterized by inflammation and high levels of eosinophils, a type of white blood cell, in the esophagus. It is a type of inflammatory bowel disease (IBD) that affects the esophagus, the muscular tube that connects the mouth to the stomach. EoE is often associated with celiac disease and type 1 diabetes, although the exact connection is still not fully understood. People with celiac disease and type 1 diabetes are more likely to develop EoE due to the impact these conditions have on the immune system. EoE can cause symptoms such as difficulty swallowing, food impaction, and heartburn. If left untreated, EoE can lead to permanent damage to the esophagus and a decrease in quality of life. Treatment for EoE typically involves a combination of dietary changes, medications, and in some cases, endoscopic procedures.

FODMAPs or Fermentable Oligosaccharides, Disaccharides, Monosaccharides and Polyols:

FODMAPs refer to a group of carbohydrates that are poorly absorbed in the small intestine, leading to fermentation in the gut and symptoms such as bloating, gas, and abdominal pain. FODMAPs include fermentable oligosaccharides (fructans and galacto-oligosaccharides), disaccharides (lactose), monosaccharides (fructose), and polyols (sugar alcohols like xylitol and sorbitol). Some common foods that contain high levels of FODMAPs include wheat, garlic, onion, apples, and dairy products.

For children with IBS or celiac disease, it is important to be mindful of their FODMAP intake, as these foods can trigger symptoms. Alternative foods that are low in FODMAPs include rice, gluten-free pasta, bananas, and potatoes. Additionally, there are many kid-friendly snack options that are naturally low in FODMAPs, such as carrots with hummus, rice crackers, and gluten-free granola bars. It is important to work with a dietitian to determine an individualized plan for managing FODMAPs, as everyone's tolerance and symptoms can vary.

Gluten:

Gluten is a type of protein found in wheat, barley, and rye that can cause an autoimmune response in individuals with celiac disease or a sensitivity to gluten. Gluten acts as a trigger for the immune system, causing it to attack the small intestine and cause damage to the villi, which are small finger-like projections in the small intestine that help absorb nutrients. This damage leads to a wide range of symptoms, including digestive issues like bloating, abdominal pain, diarrhea, and constipation.

It is important to note that gluten can hide in many unexpected places and can be present in unexpected ingredients like soy sauce, bouillon cubes, and even some medications. Additionally, gluten can also be found in processed foods like cookies, crackers, and bread. In order to avoid gluten, it is important to read food labels carefully and to be cautious about eating at restaurants, where cross-contamination with gluten can occur.

G-free or GF: Gluten-free:

"Gluten-free" refers to foods or products that do not contain any gluten, a protein found in wheat, barley, and rye. It's important to note that "gluten-free" does not always mean "gluten-free" in its truest sense. For example, some products may not contain gluten ingredients but may be processed in facilities that also process gluten-containing products, making them subject to cross-contamination.

Some naturally gluten-free foods include fresh fruits and vegetables, meat, poultry, fish, and dairy products. There are also many gluten-free snacks that are readily available, such as rice cakes, gluten-free crackers, and gluten-free granola bars. It's important for individuals with celiac disease or gluten intolerance to be vigilant about reading food labels and to be aware of hidden sources of gluten, like soy sauce and some soups and sauces.

"Honeymoon Phase":

The honeymoon phase in type 1 diabetes is a time when the body is still producing some of its own insulin. However, the levels of insulin production can be inconsistent and can lead to fluctuating needs for supplemental insulin. This can make glucose management difficult and may cause frustration for new parents managing the condition. It's important to note that these fluctuations are a normal part of the honeymoon phase and should not be seen as a reflection of the parents' efforts. Many new parents managing type 1 diabetes may feel like failures during this stage, but it's important to understand that the inconsistent insulin production is normal and not a result of their efforts or abilities.

Individualized Education Plan (IEP):

An IEP, or Individualized Education Plan, is a written document that outlines the specific educational needs of a student with disabilities and outlines the accommodations and support the school will provide to help the student succeed in the educational setting. An IEP is designed for students who require specialized instruction to meet their unique needs. This may include students with physical, cognitive, or emotional disabilities, or those with chronic health conditions such as diabetes.

The main difference between a 504 plan and an IEP is the level of support provided to the student. A 504 plan is intended to provide accommodations to students with disabilities, such as extra time on tests or the use of medical equipment in the classroom, without changing the general curriculum. On the other hand, an IEP provides specialized instruction and support, such as special education services or modifications to the curriculum, to help the student succeed.

For children with diabetes, an IEP may be necessary if their condition significantly impacts their ability to learn and participate in the educational environment. For example, a child with uncontrolled diabetes may need additional educational support to address learning gaps or mental health/counseling needs that result from their condition(s). However, for many children with diabetes, a 504 plan is often sufficient in providing the necessary accommodations, such as access to medical equipment or time for breaks to manage their condition. It is important to note that children who do not require specialized instruction and support, but simply need accommodations to manage their diabetes, are often better suited for a 504 plan rather than an IEP.

Insulin:

A hormone produced by the pancreas that regulates glucose levels in the body. In Type 1 Diabetes, the pancreas is unable to produce insulin, and thus it must be taken via injections or an insulin pump. There are different types of insulin, including rapid-acting and long-acting insulins, which are designed to mimic the body's natural insulin secretion. Fast-acting insulin is usually taken before a meal and works quickly to lower elevated blood glucose levels. Long-lasting insulin is usually taken once or twice a day and provides a constant low level of insulin to help regulate blood glucose levels throughout the day and night.

Despite popular belief, there are no herbal or naturopathic remedies that can replace insulin for those with Type 1 Diabetes.

There are several methods of insulin delivery, including syringes and needles, insulin pumps and insulin pens.

*Recently some endocrinologists have been working with Type 1 diabetics using inhaled insulins, but this is much less common in the Type 1 community.

Insulin Allergy:

Insulin allergy refers to an immune system reaction to insulin, which is the hormone responsible for regulating glucose levels in the body. There are two main types of insulin allergies: immediate and delayed. Immediate insulin allergy is a rare but severe reaction that occurs within minutes of injection and can cause symptoms like hives, itching, difficulty breathing, and low blood pressure. Delayed insulin allergy is a more common type of reaction that occurs several hours after injection and can cause symptoms like itching, redness, and swelling at the injection site.

For individuals with insulin allergies, managing their glucose levels becomes more complicated as they need to find alternative methods of insulin delivery. In some cases, they may need to switch to oral medications or insulin pumps, or even resort to alternative forms of insulin such as those made from animal sources. It's important for these individuals to work closely with their healthcare team to find the best insulin management options for their specific needs and allergies.

Insulin Pen:

This is a device used to deliver insulin to the body. It's a convenient and easy-to-use alternative to traditional insulin injections and vials. However, for young children with diabetes, administering insulin via an insulin pen can be challenging. Infants and toddlers require very small doses of insulin, which most insulin pens cannot accommodate.

Insulin Pump:

An insulin pump is a device used by individuals with Type 1 diabetes to deliver insulin into the body. It provides a continuous flow of insulin and allows for greater flexibility in insulin delivery as compared to traditional injections using a vial and syringe. The pump can be attached to the body and is typically worn 24/7.

There are different types of insulin pumps, including traditional pumps and tubeless systems. Despite its benefits, using an insulin pump can present some challenges. Accessibility can be limited in certain places, site irritation may occur, and pump failures can happen. It is important for individuals using an insulin pump to have a backup plan and know how to use a traditional vial and syringe system to administer insulin in case of pump failure, shortage of supplies or other emergency situations.

Intravenous (IV):

An IV is a medical procedure where a catheter is inserted into a vein in order to provide fluids, medications, or nutrition directly into the bloodstream. In severe cases of diabetic ketoacidosis (DKA), the body becomes dehydrated, which can cause veins to become small or collapse. This makes it difficult to insert an IV line in the traditional arm veins. In these cases, the healthcare provider may use alternative placement methods, such as the scalp vein or jugular vein, to insert the IV line. These alternative placement methods allow for the rapid administration of fluids and insulin, which are essential in treating DKA.

J1:

A J1 school diet accommodation refers to a special diet that is provided to a student with a medical condition, such as diabetes or celiac disease, in order to meet their dietary needs while they are at school. This accommodation is often outlined in a 504 plan and allows the student to have access to appropriate foods and snacks throughout the school day to maintain their health and support their diabetes management. The J1 accommodation is a way for schools to ensure that students with medical conditions are able to participate fully in school activities and not be discriminated against or excluded because of their dietary requirements.

MDI: Multiple Daily Injections:

A method of delivering insulin using syringes or insulin pens. This method is considered to be the most basic and widely available method of insulin delivery and is often the first method recommended for newly diagnosed individuals. The reason for this is that it provides the user with more control over the amount of insulin being delivered and helps them to better understand the action and absorption of insulin in their body.

MDI requires the combined use of long and fast-acting insulins. It involves injecting long-lasting insulin 1-2 times per day and fast-acting insulin several times a day before meals and snacks, or to correct high blood glucose levels throughout the day. The frequency and amount of injections will depend on the individual's needs and the recommendations of their doctor. MDI is often considered a flexible and cost-effective method of insulin delivery, making it a popular option for many people with Type 1 Diabetes.

NPO or "Nothing by Mouth":

In medical terms, NPO is an order given to patients to refrain from consuming food or drink, typically for a specific period of time. When it comes to diabetes, NPO is often used for individuals who have been newly diagnosed with DKA (Diabetic Ketoacidosis) and are admitted to the hospital.

Additionally, NPO status is important to avoid further taxing the body and potentially triggering any additional complications. Individuals with DKA may have elevated insulin needs and taking in food or drink could lead to further instability in their blood glucose levels. Keeping individuals NPO helps to minimize the risk of any further complications and provides the best chance for a full recovery.

Pancreas:

The pancreas is a gland located in the abdomen that plays a crucial role in regulating blood sugar levels. It produces insulin, a hormone that helps the body's cells absorb glucose (sugar) from the bloodstream to use as energy. In individuals with Type 1 diabetes, the pancreas is unable to produce insulin due to the destruction of the insulin-producing cells (beta cells) in the pancreas. This results in high levels of glucose in the blood, which can lead to various health problems if not properly managed through insulin injections or an insulin pump. In individuals with Type 2 diabetes, the pancreas may still produce insulin, but the cells in the body become resistant to its effects. This leads to a decreased ability of the insulin to effectively regulate blood sugar levels, leading to elevated glucose levels. The role of the pancreas in diabetes highlights the importance of maintaining healthy pancreatic function for overall health and well-being.

Pancreatic Transplant:

A pancreatic transplant is a surgical procedure where a healthy pancreas from a donor is implanted into a person with diabetes. The main purpose of this transplant is to replace the damaged or non-functioning pancreas, which is responsible for producing insulin, a hormone that regulates blood sugar levels in the body.

Currently, pancreatic transplantation is considered a high-risk procedure, with many potential complications, including rejection of the transplanted organ, bleeding, infection, and problems with the blood supply to the new pancreas. Despite these risks, some people with diabetes choose to undergo the procedure because it has the potential to cure their diabetes, eliminate the need for insulin injections, and improve overall health.

To date, thousands of pancreatic transplants have been performed worldwide, with varying success rates. However, this procedure is still considered experimental, and it is only recommended for people with severe and uncontrolled diabetes. After the transplant, the recipient must take powerful immunosuppressant drugs to prevent the body from rejecting the new pancreas, which can increase the risk of infection and other health problems.

While pancreatic transplantation has shown promise in the management of diabetes, it is not a cure-all. The procedure is still in the early stages of development, and more research is needed to determine its long-term benefits and risks. However, for some people with diabetes, it may be a viable option to help improve their quality of life and manage their condition more effectively.

T1D: Type 1 Diabetes:

Type 1 Diabetes is an autoimmune disease in which the body's immune system attacks and destroys the beta cells in the pancreas, which produce insulin. Unlike Type 2 Diabetes, Type 1 Diabetes is not caused by poor diet or lifestyle habits. Instead, it is a genetic condition that affects individuals from all walks of life, regardless of their diet, exercise habits, or weight. This condition is most commonly diagnosed in children and young adults, and it requires daily management through insulin injections or an insulin pump to regulate blood glucose levels. There is currently no cure for Type

1 Diabetes, and individuals with this condition must rely on insulin for the rest of their lives to stay healthy and manage their blood glucose levels.

T2D: Type 2 Diabetes:

Type 2 Diabetes is a chronic condition that affects the way the body processes insulin and glucose. Unlike Type 1 Diabetes, which is an autoimmune condition, Type 2 Diabetes is often the result of a combination of genetic and lifestyle factors. However, despite these differences, there is still a significant amount of stigma surrounding both types of diabetes. People with Type 2 Diabetes are often thought to have caused their condition through poor diet and lifestyle habits, leading to hurtful assumptions and discrimination. These assumptions are not only incorrect, but they can also be damaging to an individual's self-esteem and mental health. It's important to understand that both Type 1 and Type 2 Diabetes are serious conditions that require proper management and support. Individuals with either type of diabetes should not be judged or stigmatized based on their condition.

IBS/Irritable Bowel Syndrome:

IBS is a gastrointestinal disorder that affects the large intestine. It is characterized by symptoms such as abdominal pain, bloating, constipation, and diarrhea. IBS is a common condition that is often associated with celiac disease. People with celiac disease have an autoimmune reaction to gluten, which is a protein found in wheat, barley, and rye. This autoimmune response can cause damage to the small intestine, leading to the development of IBS symptoms. In fact, it is estimated that up to 25% of people with celiac disease also have IBS. This is because the damage caused by the autoimmune response can affect the digestive system, leading to symptoms such as abdominal pain, bloating, and diarrhea. It's important for individuals with celiac disease to maintain a strict gluten-free diet in order to manage both their celiac symptoms and any IBS symptoms that may arise.

References

The following is a list of resources (some quite formal and academic, others less so). There are a few narrative works, like this one on the list, but not many, because they just don't seem to exist. It is my hope that more will enter the landscape over time.

Bliss, Michael. The Discovery of Insulin. Chicago: U of Chicago, 1982. Print.

Bradley, James. "The Surprising Things Doctors Learned by Tasting Patients' Urine." PostEverything. The Washington Post, 11 July 2014. Web. 20 Mar. 2016.

Breecher, Maury M., and Tim Anderson. "Frederick Banting, MD." Science Heroes. Holdings Inc., n.d. Web. Mar. 2016.

Bzowyckyj, A., & Stahnke, A. (2018). "Hypersensitivity reactions to human insulin analogs in insulin-naïve patients: a systematic review." Therapeutic Advances in Endocrinology and Metabolism, 9(2): 53–65.

Cooper, Thea, and Arthur Ainsberg. Breakthrough. New York: St. Martins, 2010. Print.

Dorn, C. Public Posting. Facebook, 4 December, 2019.

Heinzerling, L., Raile, K., Rochlitz, H., Zuberbier, M., & Worm, M. (2008). "Insulin Allergy: Clinical Manifestations and Management Strategies

Hirsch, I. B. "History of Glucose Monitoring." University of Washington.

Hirsch, James. "The Durable Diabetic: Gladys Dull Relies on the Basics to Make Medial

History." DiaTribe. The DiaTribe Foundation, 07 June 2007. Web. 25. 2016.

Maahs, David M., et al. "Insulin Pump Use by Children is Highest in US, Collaboration Found." TID Exchange. National Paediatric Diabetes Audit and the Royal College of Paediatrics and Child Health Registries, 10. Nov. 2014. Web. 16 Feb. 2016.

Petersen, C. "Are Divorce Rates Really Higher for Families With Special Needs Kids?" Parent.com. 25 January 2018.

Prentice, Ann. "Constituents of Human Milk." Food and Nutrition Bulletin 17:4. United Nations University, Dec. 1996. Web. 10 Aug. 2014.

Redd, Nola T. "Apollo 11: First Men on the Moon." Space.com. Purch, 25 July 2012. Web. 25 Mar. 2016.

Science News (2012). "90th Anniversary Issue: 1970s." 181.6 (2012): 28. Society for Science and the Public. Web. 25 Mar. 2016.

Seward, Zacharay M. "The First Mobile Phone Call Was Made 40 Years Ago Today." The Atlantic. Atlantic Media Company, 3 Apr. 2013. Web. 25 Mar. 2016.

Sheehan, Mar. Elle & Coach. Hatchett Books. 2016.

Sobsey, Dick. "Marital Stability and Marital Satisfaction in Families of Children with Disabilities: Chicken or Egg?" Developmental Disabilities Bulletin 32.1 (2004): 62-83. University of Alberta. Web.

Tattersall, Robert. Diabetes: The Biography. Oxford: Oxford UP, 2009. Print.

Turner, Jim. "Novo Story of Insulin." DLife. 1 Feb. 2010. YouTube. Web. 25 Mar.

Other Books By This Author

Erin also writes kid-friendly titles that feature positive diabetes representation.

Nonfiction: *Get to Know Frederick Banting*

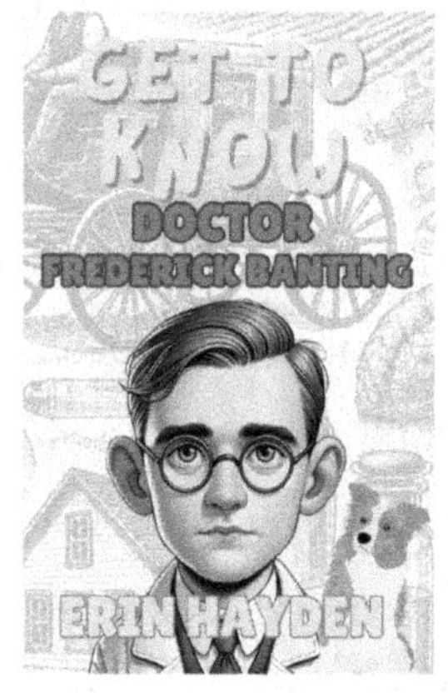

Get ready to embark on an incredible journey through the life of Frederick Banting—a true hero who did it all! In this fascinating nonfiction book, you'll discover the remarkable story of Frederick Banting, who was a medical researcher and so much more! He was also a brave war hero and a talented painter. But he was also a complex person with worries and faults, just like everyone else.

Frederick's journey starts on a quiet farm in a small town in Canada, where he learned the value of hard work and responsibility. But as he grew up, he dreamed of doing something bigger than running the farm like his family wanted him to do. Along the way, he faced incredible challenges, like failing in his first year of college and surviving World War I.

Frederick's life was far from ordinary. He didn't just become a doctor--he became a medical pioneer! He discovered how to make insulin, a life-saving medicine for people with diabetes. Can you believe it? His work changed the world has saved millions of lives over the past 100 years.

This book will take you on an adventure, filled with stories of courage, discovery, and the power of never giving up. Frederick Banting's life is a testament to what one person can achieve with determination and a heart full of compassion. Get ready to be inspired by this incredible man who made the world a better place.

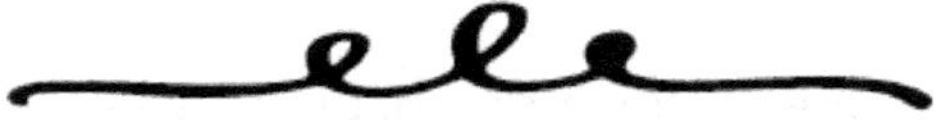

Fiction Series: *The Sugar Squad Chronicles*

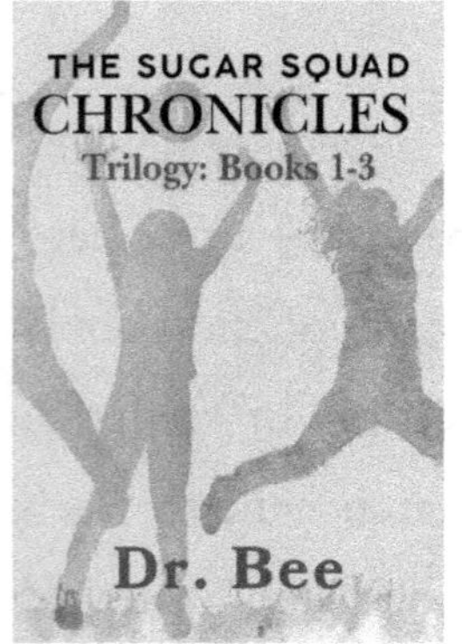

Join the adventures of friends Ava and Grayson in The Sugar Squad Chronicles, an awesome new series full of laughs and mystery!

In Book 1: *Camp Lessons*, the adventure begins when Ava and Grayson meet at summer diabetes camp. They bond over hiking, cooking, and reeling the biggest catfish the camp has ever seen! The fun continues with campfires, memory-book making and epic stories from motorcycle-riding Nurse Sean. But the action doesn't end when camp does.

Through Ava and Grayson's eyes, this collection helps raise awareness about important health issues like diabetes and celiac disease while weaving in universal themes of friendship, adventure, and resilience. With a dynamic mix of mystery, adventure, and even a dash of danger, these stories offer a vibrant backdrop for exploring real-world challenges like bullying and family separation. As the squad gains members in each book, this tight-knit group discovers that teamwork triumphs over any obstacle. And in Book 3, A Sweetwater Mystery, the fate of the camp is at stake—The Squad will need to work together to crack the case!

With enduring friendships and page-turning suspense, you'll be rooting for these brave heroes and want to join their Squad yourself!

Chronicles Series, Book 4: *A Road Trip Adventure*

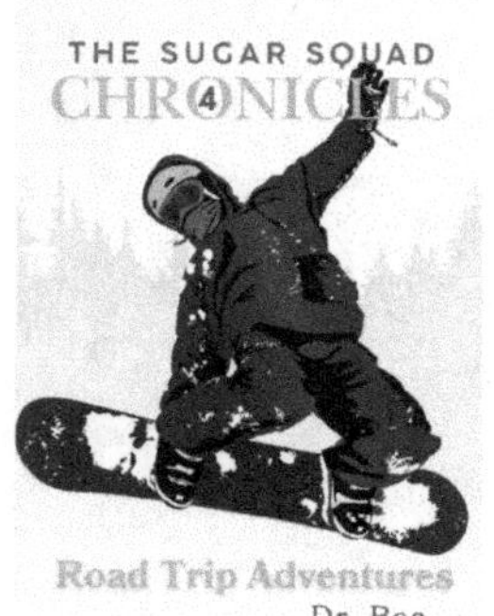

Grayson is in for the road trip of a lifetime when his family heads across the Southwest visiting auto-tech programs for big brother Hunter. Missing his friends back home, Grayson is happily surprised by a special encounter midway through the journey. And a few epic snowboarding adventures don't hurt either!

But this once-in-a-lifetime road trip is threatened with an abrupt ending when brother Hunter falls ill. Confronted with evil stories of the past and an unsettling trend of missing girls on his friend Lilly's reservation, Grayson may have gotten more than he bargained for with this trip.

Armed with optimism and bravery, Grayson and his Squad swiftly hatch a plan to combat the evil threatening Lilly, but soon discover that some problems are too complicated for kids alone to fix.

Follow along on another bumpy adventure with the Sugar Squad, where innocence and harsh reality sometimes collide. Using tight bonds and humor when hope seems lost, these everyday heroes discover how to balance childhood dreams with grownup challenges, one day at a time.

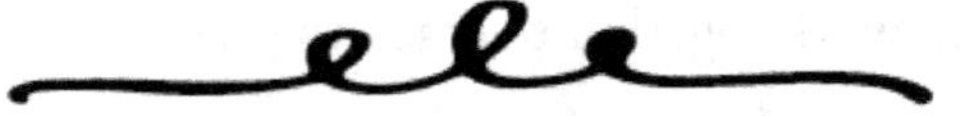

If You Enjoyed This Book

If you enjoyed reading this story and would like to see more like it, please help me share this book with others.

Here are some ways you can help other kids learn about this book:

Leave a review on your favorite book retail or review platform:

- Review Tip: Your review doesn't have to be long. One or two sentences is great!

- Vote Up: If you see other reviews that you think are helpful, you can click the little "Helpful" box to give them a boost.

Tell your friends, family and anyone else you can think of:

- Do you belong to a book club? Great news—this newest edition of the book comes complete with discussion questions!

- Ask your local library or small bookstore to add this book to their collection. I'd be happy to come for a Meet the Author event!

Contact Me! I love and reply to all fan-mail!

- Email: Erin@BraveryBooks.com

- Join my newsletter where you can stay up to date on new releases (for both kids and adults!).

- Book a speaking event: Would you like me to come speak at your library or local bookstore? Email me at Erin@BraveryBooks.com to make arrangements.

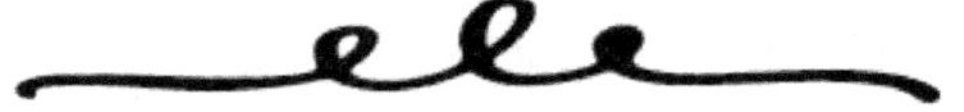

Book Club Discussion Questions

1. As mothers, we all want to believe "this could never happen to my child." How did reading these stories reshape your definition of "normal" childhood?

2. These moms often felt crushed by guilt over "failing" their child somehow. Could you relate to those unrelenting feelings of guilt for things that were actually out of your control?

3. Was there a scene in the book that made you think, "I don't know how she does it!" Can you relate to feelings of being completely overwhelmed yet pushing through?

4. Managing complex care while running a household is an incredible feat! Did these stories make you appreciate or think differently about the division of duties in your own home?

5. Be honest - did parts of this book terrify you as a parent? Were there moments that made you want to hug your own child a little

tighter or feel grateful for their health?

6. We saw mothers fighting rigid hospital policies, especially when trying to continue nursing their young children after diagnosis. Why do you think abrupt weaning would have been so traumatic that these mothers felt the need to push back?

7. We all judge mom-moments through our own personal lens! Were there any decisions by these mothers that made you think, "Oh honey, I would NOT have done that!"?

8. If facing a crisis like the diagnosis of a young child with a chronic illness, do you think your social circle would step up? Who in your life could you absolutely count on?

9. Advancements in diabetes management now help individuals live long and active lives. What past scenarios shocked you? Were there any challenges that still exist today that you found surprising?

10. What do you think about the potential of an ordeal like this to make or break a marriage? Would facing something similar strengthen or strain your own relationship?

www.ingramcontent.com/pod-product-compliance
Lightning Source LLC
LaVergne TN
LVHW050539160826
845677LV00011B/2092
9798230181316